AFFECTION

an erotic memoir

KRISSY KNEEN

SEAL PRESS

AFFECTION
an erotic memoir

Copyright © 2010 by Krissy Kneen

Published by
Seal Press
A Member of the Perseus Books Group
1700 Fourth Street
Berkeley, California

Library of Congress Cataloging-in-Publication Data

Kneen, Krissy, 1968-
  Affection : an erotic memoir / Krissy Kneen.
    p. cm.
  ISBN 978-1-58005-342-6
  1. Kneen, Krissy, 1968—Sexual behavior. 2. Women—Sexual behavior—Australia. I. Title.
  HQ29.K59 2010
  306.77092—dc22
  [B]
                        2010014521

9 8 7 6 5 4 3 2 1

Cover and interior design by Domini Dragoone
Printed in the United States of America by Edwards Brothers
Distributed by Publishers Group West

In order to protect the identities of those people who were kind enough to share their stories to benefit the reader, many names have been changed.

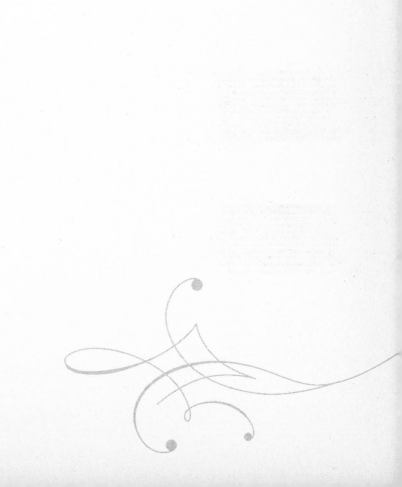

CONTENTS

BOUND

Richard tied me to a pole because I asked him to. He used duct tape and he secured my wrists with it. The mattress was within reach but only close enough to rest my head on. He tied a sock around my face; I could still see if I opened my eyes and squinted. The floor was concrete and I felt the chill bite of it in my knees. He had tied my hands low, and I could stand but not straighten. Kneeling was best, my head resting on the pillow of my bound palms. My back arched up, my bottom raised. I knew where this was leading.

There was something strangely domestic about the morning. He filled the sink and I could hear the clatter of plates in the soapy water. Upstairs a similar scene was in progress, our landlady washing her own dishes, a domestic parallel minus the girl tied to the pole in the middle of the room.

I imagined that he would look up from the dishes and watch me. I wondered if I looked ridiculous in submission, if he was grinning with the humor of it all. Perhaps he watched impassively, clocking the time by the fading heat of the water. I heard him empty the sink and fill it again. Time passing. The slow drip of dishes drying. The television upstairs chattering about nothing to no one.

My skin became my eyes. I felt the fingers growing out of my back, wriggling like an anemone, my tentacles of awareness picking out small changes in the breeze and temperature. If someone had photographed me like this there would have been a hazy outline. Kirlian photography would have captured the little bubble of awareness that enveloped me. I thought about the boy upstairs, Richard's previous lover. The boy upstairs watching football on television as his mother did the dishes, and in the downstairs parallel universe my lover—his ex-lover—and me, tied to the pole.

I grew restless. I wanted to call him over to me. I wanted his hands and his body and some relief from this stretching out of my skin. I imagine that he spent an age over the drying because he wanted me to enjoy my time of longing, but I am not sure I enjoyed the long minutes of waiting. When he came to me finally, I could have ripped the duct tape off the pole and finished in a second but I did nothing. Said nothing.

He examined me. I felt his hands still dripping with dishwashing liquid, lifting, pulling, separating. Of course I knew how this would end, but still there was the little shivery thrill as he traced the ridge of bone arcing down from the center of my back, slipping his finger over, but not into, my anus, and hooking it into my vagina, testing the viscosity there.

I thought of dissection tables, dead things tied down, paws and legs splayed, bellies exposed to the glare of fluorescent light. The fact that this aroused me was perhaps a problem. The erotic appeal of the medical experiment had become a recurring theme.

It was the idea of him watching me like that, the openness, the vulnerability. There was no question that he would penetrate me eventually, but he took his time. The joy is not knowing exactly when, and exactly where. The joy is the anticipation. A moment of breath on the skin, a sense of exposure, a vulnerability. Someone watching or not watching; never knowing which. I remember the hot cold of the afternoon and the disappointment of the inevitable ending. The sound of his ex-boyfriend turning off the television at the moment of his orgasm, a sudden silence and the slight, pleasurable pain of his withdrawal. The normalcy of a Sunday morning creeping into afternoon.

I will always remember this, perhaps. I remember it now.

And that was just the sex part.

SEX ADDICTION

Brisbane 2008

"Sex addict?" I laugh. "I'm not a sex addict."

Katherine raises an eyebrow. I have known her since I was eighteen. She is the friend who has stuck by me longest. I look at her gorgeous luminous face and I wonder why we have never slept together, not once in all these years. She sips at her coffee and watches me and I feel myself unpicked; and when I am seamless there is nothing left of me but sex. I have been pathologized.

I picture an ape, furiously masturbating in its enclosure; I can feel the ugly monkey suit itching against my skin and for a brief moment I am repelled and also aroused by the image. I am used to this sudden rush of desire, the narcotic effect of the idea of sex, a prickly spread of it like ecstasy trickling through my body.

I am made of sex, I feed on the thought of it. I call myself Queer because there is no other word I know to describe this state of being indiscriminately sexual. Now Katherine has made new words for me to worry over. Sex addict. An addiction.

I would like to tell her that I'm not addicted, that I could stop any time. It would be a joke and it would also be untrue.

A young Asian man walks into the café and I glance at him and register his feminine beauty. Again the rush of pleasure. That comforting settling low in my belly. There was a time when I would have made some kind of contact with this man, slipped over to his table, engaged in some light flirtation; heavier if he responded. There was a time when we might have ended up in bed together.

"If I am an addict then I have got it under control."

"How many times a day do you think about sex?"

Almost constantly.

"How often do you masturbate?"

I sigh. She knows that I can never stay alone in the house if I am to get any work done at all. She knows that I struggle not to look up pornography on the Internet. She knows me almost as well as I know myself.

"Heaps of people think about sex as much as I do. Men. I am just a man trapped inside a woman's body." A throwaway line, and she laughs.

"Teenage boys, perhaps. You are going to be forty this year."

I shrug.

"How many shrinks does it take to change a lightbulb?"

"Well yes." She smiles at the old joke that has lasted between us through all the years. "There is the question of whether the lightbulb wants to change."

I hold her delicate fingers and smile, and I think about how deeply she could reach inside me with those elegant hands. A wriggling fish of thought, fleeting, gone in a second, but there will be another and another, whole schools of thought flashing across my consciousness. The constant distractions of a sexual world as wonderful and varied as the ocean, a world I could drown myself in and die happy.

"I don't think I'm a sex addict." I check my watch. Just enough time to catch a bus to work.

We stand and hug and there is her willowy body pressed against mine for just a moment. I rarely hug. Hugs are an open doorway to a flaring in my body and I remove myself from these kinds of intimate gestures. No hugging, no kisses on the cheek, no holding hands unless I feel safe enough with the person I am touching.

I hug Katherine, my oldest friend, who has just now pinned me with her observation.

"You take care," she tells me, and she means it. She always wishes me well. I watch her walking away from me, graceful, slender, the line of her perfect breasts under a tight sweater, and that liquid surge pumps through my brain. I am, of course, not a sex addict, but as I watch her walk away from me, feeding on my lust as if it were a Lindt ball dissolving under my tongue, I pause, and I wonder.

CHILDHOOD

Blacktown 1970

The wonderful thing about felt pictures is the way you can rub them on your upper lip and they feel like comfort. They are simple shapes cut out of bright colors. The felt sticks to itself with a satisfying grab. If you get very close all the colors blend into each other and the shapes disappear. A horse is no longer a horse. A house is not a house.

I have become obsessive about felt pictures. I lie on the scratchy carpet, pushing my body down against the short pile. The television is on, *Playschool* or *Mr. Squiggle* or *Bill and Ben the Flowerpot Men* or some other burble of music and rhyme. My hips press against the carpet and the delightful pressure of a full bladder, full of milk no doubt, a lovely innocent pressure and the feel of sunlight burning a window shape on my calves. Red horse, orange horse, yellow, all of a palette. I save the blues and greens for the other corner of the felt board. I hoard fish and crabs and grass and green houses for the cool color end of things. I am sleepy and the colors blend into each other. They blend into the throb of my bladder and when I cross my legs over each other there is an even greater pleasure. I can hear my mother clattering through the washing up.

Color. I see color. I feel heat and pressure and the edges of everything become indistinct. I hover at the edge of a thought. Perhaps I will fall asleep midhorse. I arrange the horses one next to another next to another. All the orange horses. Perhaps I will just let go, urinate ecstatically on the scratchy carpet. The pressure builds, my eyelids droop, I see orange and red and there is a smell to it, a burnt caramel sweetness and I breathe in deeply, wondering what it could be.

When I fall over the edge I am surprised. Pleased. It is as if I have succumbed to color. I am filled with it, and full of the idea of smell. My skin is burning with all kinds of blue. The down on the back of my neck is sweet as honey. My body pulses in the aftermath of this transformation.

This was my first orgasm. I can name it now. I can relive it. But back then, at the beginning of things, there was no line between the colors and the heat and the scent. After this moment I fell in love with the process of making pictures with felt. I came back to this activity again and again and again and again. Felt pictures first and then, when my mother thought I was old enough, oil paints meted out onto the upturned lid of a margarine container.

"Not too much linseed oil."

The oil thinned the color, made it slick and shiny, thin on the canvas. The oil painting was something we did together, my mother and I. My sister was too fiercely independent to sit and listen to instruction. She was naturally talented. She painted horses and dragons and princesses. She made paper dolls for me to play with and the most elaborate dresses painted on cartridge paper. Little paper tabs to fold over the bare shoulders of the beautiful paper women.

I painted till my body hummed with color. I pressed my knees together and breathed in the heady scent of turpentine till my head began to spin. I didn't know about sex but I knew that I should never tell about the thing the colors did to my body. I lay under a blanket and turned the thick glossy pages of an art book. Chagall blue, my favorite color in the world, and my fist pressed firmly against my pubis. Blue and pleasure, that was all there was to the world until my sister ripped the blanket from my body and left me exposed to the bare gray light of the day.

"I know what you're doing," she chanted. "I know, I know, I know."

But I didn't know.

No one spoke to me about masturbation. I didn't know that what I did had anything to do with sex. I didn't know that people touched each other to make this happen without the smell of paint and the vision of color.

My house was sexless. There were five industrious women, and my grandfather hiding invisible in his room. My grandmother sat above us like a queen bee and the rest of the women listened and obeyed. My father was absent. My sister says I should remember the presence of my father, but it is gone as if the short time he was with me in childhood has been erased. That part of the tape was exposed to a magnet or the sun.

When I discovered the physical way of achieving orgasm, the full knowledge that certain pressures of my fingers would produce such an overwhelmingly pleasurable result, I could not stop doing it. I became an expert at it, finding places that would be private, times when I could sneak away and would not be missed.

Bath times, quick trips to the toilet, and in the evenings, drowsy from the day.

I shared a room with my sister and I practiced staying awake till I was certain that she would be asleep. I was stealthy as a ninja, one finger rubbing so gently that the bed wouldn't even creak. On the weekend I could sometimes find a quiet spot, private, secluded. There was a crawl space beside the house, overgrown with jasmine and gated by two gardenia bushes pressing their branches together. This was my favorite place, the summer scent, perfumes clamoring, the fat buzz of bees droning sleepy in my ear.

I pulled down my shirt, exposing my shoulders to the scratch of leaves and the finger creep of a lazy breeze. I imagined I was naked. I hadn't even taken my knickers all the way off. I pulled them to one side and they were a damp obstruction to be worked around. There would be grass in my hair, twin plaits, all that wiriness pulled tight. My skirt would suck the damp from the soil. I would be in disarray when I pushed my way back into the world, blinking at the slap of sunlight. There was no other human being in my imaginings. There was just the sense of all the elements settling on my flesh. The scent alone whispered love. White flowers, sharp and sweeter than honey, a drugged haze of scent pulling me down. There was the Chagall blue behind my closed eyelids. When my mother called I was a long way away, drifting toward a precipice without hurry. With the sound of her voice I was rushing, scared by the possibility of discovery. The fear was a kind of excitement, hurrying toward a quick, barely satisfying climax. I dug my fingers into the soil, masking the smell of my juices with earthworm castings and loamy grit.

THE BOOKSHOP

Brisbane 2008

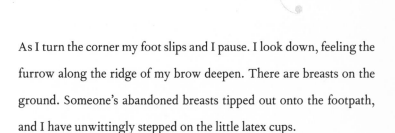

As I turn the corner my foot slips and I pause. I look down, feeling the furrow along the ridge of my brow deepen. There are breasts on the ground. Someone's abandoned breasts tipped out onto the footpath, and I have unwittingly stepped on the little latex cups.

I take out my phone and clear a space, deleting photographs of rotting fish and weed and the flash of a salmon jumping. I aim the camera and snap them up. Two perfect breasts, nipples kissing the dirty concrete, their lurid pink cups scooping sunlight out of the air.

I am early for work. Someone has slept on the gay and lesbian street press leaving a nest of paper and a scattering of crumbs in the door-way. There are locks and bolts to open, bending, standing, reaching. My morning workout. There is a new lock for every time the shop has been burgled. Nothing deters the thieves but we seem to feel safer the more keys we have to carry.

I lock the door behind me and breathe in the dust of five thousand books. I have a habit of checking in with my favorite authors when I arrive. I touch the shelves. O is for Ondaatje, C is for Crace, D is for Delillo and Donovan.

I stash my bag on top of the pile of unidentifiable crap in the cupboard and punch the code for the safe. Money in the tills, lights on, the terrible sinking sensation of another day all set up and ready to begin.

I take my phone out and scroll through the photographs until I find the one I am looking for, a pair of silicone breasts abandoned on the footpath. In the photograph the breasts are upturned, their nipples grazing the pavement. I should have turned them up the other way. It is perhaps a little difficult to identify them in their upturned pose. I am still quite early for work; there is time to rectify the photograph but that would ruin the spontaneity of the thing.

Key in the door. Christopher lifts a hand in greeting. "Morning," and he lumbers over to the cupboard and throws his backpack onto the top of the pile.

"Sleeping in the doorway again Krissy?"

"As always."

I read Christopher's story this morning and it was heartbreaking. It was so fine and pure and beautiful that I wanted it to be about me. He has decided to write a story a day and I am quietly jealous of his commitment and his talent. He is fifteen years younger than me and he has become my hero. I almost hate him for it.

"I stepped on a pair of breasts today," I tell him and he nods and makes no comment. It has been years since my observations caused any reaction in him. He has settled into the routine of working alongside me, glancing past my outrageous statements and flirtatious manner. He has grown fond of me, but I am taken for granted. This is the story of my life. And it is getting worse. More than ever now I am left to wait at a counter while the shop assistant serves the younger customers, the prettier customers, the taller customers.

Christopher bends toward the safe and I could stop him; I have already removed the money, there is nothing to find there, but I watch him bend, the bottom of his jacket riding up, exposing a soft expanse of creamy flesh that looks almost edible. I think of crème brûlée, custard, something sweet and rich.

"I've got the cash out already." I tell him this too late. I could have saved him the bend and stretch, but it was a good moment and I savor the quick visual rush. I think about what Katherine has said. An addiction. My day is ripe with little moments like this, morsels of desire measured out through the otherwise empty hours. I snack on my little desires and I am never too full for another bite.

I watch as Christopher struggles back to standing. He is too close and I step back. I feign lazy indifference to his solid height, the scent of soap and hint of sweat. I am fleetingly appalled at myself. An addiction. But surely I have it under control.

I flip open my phone and scroll down to the photograph. "Look."

"You really meant it. Breasts."

I nod.

"I thought you were being metaphorical."

"How do you metaphorically step on a pair of breasts?"

He takes the phone out of my hand and our fingers brush lightly, again that electric current of flesh on flesh. I am a detonator, rattled by every little touch or glance or anonymous passing by, but I have begun to notice Christopher more often than not. It is something about his writing and our friendship. It has begun to trouble me.

Christopher hands me the phone and turns back toward the tills. "I don't know, I thought it was just one of your sex things."

He empties the change into the drawers. I try not to watch him.

"There's more to me than just sex things," I tell him.

He snorts as if I am making a joke. "I wonder who lost their breasts," he says, rattling coins and pulling bills out of a tight roll. "How do you lose your breasts like that?"

I check my watch. Time to open the shop. We struggle to move the card table with its spill of sale books, the A-frame board, the easel. He presses play on the CD. I prepare myself for a day electric with interactions. A critical mass of flesh easing in and out of the shop, men and women who love to read. Warm bodies in a tryst with literature.

"Okay," says Christopher, standing too close, "I'm going upstairs to do my ordering. You okay with it? Call me if you need a hand." He eases away and I relax again. Of course I have always been a ball of pent-up desire; but I won't thank Katherine for pointing it out to me in such clinical terms. An addiction. A sexual addiction.

An older woman wanders through the children's section. I hover nearby, I smile.

"Do you need a hand finding something?" I ask, and I notice how clear and intelligent her eyes are. I notice her perfume and her elegantly wrinkled hands, her grace and her warmth and—yes, Katherine, I think I might actually have a problem.

PAPIER-MÂCHÉ

Blacktown 1977

We are not a family who works at remembering. There are my grandmother's childhood stories and these are more complete and vivid than
any of our own. We remember her father who liked to make shoes and
tell her stories. We remember her aunt who dropped a heavy tray on
her cousin's head from a great height. We remember her train ride to
safety, alone and frightened and chilled by icy winds. Collectively,
our family remembers the heat of Egypt, the grit of sand in our teeth,
the little boys with flies sipping from their sweaty eyelids.

In my grandmother's kitchen we ate fulmedames and vegetables stuffed with rice. Gnocchi that she had painstakingly rolled out
on a folding card table in front of daytime movies filmed in Italian
and badly dubbed into English. I watched her lips move as she followed them and wondered what language she was hearing inside her

head. My grandmother's cooking was a haphazard mix of Egyptian meals and European dishes. When pressed, she was always cryptic about her heritage.

"I come from no man's land," she told us, her accent harsh and jagged, Germanic crispness, a Russian flaring of the vowel sounds.

"What do you mean, no man's land?"

"There is a war and this bit," her hands portioning out the air like the dough she kneaded and tore into little buns each morning, "this bit goes to one side of this argument. This bit goes to the other." She indicated the space between the invisible territories that had been separated. "This is the no man's land. This is where I come from. Where you have to sneak things across this land that everyone is arguing about."

My mother and my aunt were born in Egypt and they sometimes talked of pyramids and the desert and the English school where they learned to speak as if they were living with the Queen. Clear crisp sentences. Exact language. I recognized this kind of studied English in the mouths of the Indian kids at school. More English than the English. In Blacktown it was an accent that could get your turban torn from your head, your head flushed down the toilet, your schoolbooks ripped into fragments and scattered down Flushcombe Road.

Of my own childhood, there is barely anything left. I remember moments of it with photographic clarity, events that stand out from the general ravage of years, but the rest is all old bone, barely recognizable. In the void I reach for fragments. Scraps of abandoned play: jumping over an obstacle course in a pony-canter, rolling in mud till there is nothing left of my skin, peppering my clothing with the slow lumber and drag of snails, watching a silver lacework form in their slimy paths. I smell gardenia and orange blossom and honeysuckle and every memory is infused with a postcoital languidness. Childhood is fat and lazy with the pleasures of the flesh. Everything tasted, everything held to my nose, everything rubbed against my upper lip.

In the evenings we made models together. Models that would be displayed in the museum or in libraries. This was the family trade, and I was born to be apprenticed to it. We sat out on the patio and the women smoked, lighting one cigarette off the next, their cigarette holders caked with sticky white glue. It was my job to tear the paper into even strips. Newspaper and thick slabs of telephone directories, gleaned from the post office or from neighboring houses. We needed a great deal of paper because the things we made were large.

We were working on dinosaurs at that time. They were life-sized, destined to sit in the museum when they were done, but for now they were in pieces. There were heads and torsos and clawed dinosaur arms on every chair. The dogs paced distractedly around them, trying to find enough floor space to coil their bodies into. There were dinosaur books spread out on every flat surface and the women kept checking back, coating their pages with what they called "the horrible glue."

I listened to the stories and tore paper until the boxes were filled with uniformly sized strips. The next job was to roll some of the strips into little balls, dimples that would be stuck to the surface of the brontosaurus. There was a plan for this. Dimples first, then the spongy packing foam torn into rough strips to hide the hard line of the edges, overlapping so that the dinosaur skin would look soft and pliable. My aunt was making teeth out of papier-mâché, a wire trailing out of each one so that it could easily be fixed into the toothless jaw when it was done. She dipped each tooth into a smooth plaster mix and hung it on a rack to dry.

There was intense seriousness in the detail. They took time over the faces in particular. The creases in the surface around the eyes. If the creature's expression was unconvincing my grandmother would take its whole head apart, slip the papier-mâché eyeball out and reshape it before assembling the head and reattaching it.

I recognized this kind of monofocus from my own experiences with paint. I wondered if the three of them experienced the same kind of physical rush when they were carefully moulding the papier-mâché strips onto their wire-and-wood armatures.

The smell of the glue was intoxicating. The glue and smooth skin of plaster or latex, the cans of spray paint that would be the first layer of color, the little pots of enamel paint for fine work. There were plastic bags filled with human hair waiting for the next project—Sleeping Beauty, the Little Match Girl, fairy tale princesses with each delicate eyelash cut to size and glued in place.

The women dipped their strips of paper into jars of paste, smoothed and placed them, reached inside the boxes for more paper. They never once looked up or around. They could work for hours, finally stretching up to stand in the early hours of the morning, their backs cracking.

"Enough for now," my grandmother would say in her thick Slavic accent. "For now, enough." And, as if a signal had been sounded, the rest of us would scurry to pack up the debris, lifting the dinosaur by its sturdy legs and maneuvering it into the lounge room, putting lids on the bottles of wood glue, stuffing fur fabric back into garbage bags. My family would be exhausted from long hours of complete focus but they would be happy, serenely happy. No hugs goodnight. Never a hug goodnight. Just a quick slap on the rump from my grandmother to let us know that we had done well, worked hard, achieved what she expected of us. She would never praise our work. She would nod and say, "You are my granddaughter. You will be the best. Not second place, not almost best. Top of the class."

The days were warm. There was school, but when we were not at school there was play or there was a disappearing into fiction. I remember characters in novels I was reading as if they were friends. I pick up a children's book and read a paragraph, and I smell coffee brewed in a pot on the stove and eaten with chunks of buttery homemade bread.

In my first year of school they did IQ testing. They tallied the results of the test and offered me a special sponsored place in a school for smart kids in the northern suburbs. My grandmother would not have me put in a special school like a performing monkey, she raged; I would have no social skills, locked away with the smart kids. But really I knew it was because there was already talk of me becoming a boarder. The commute from Blacktown to the North Shore would be too arduous; I could not do it alone. And there would be boys at the school. I would be alone with boys, and perhaps male teachers. We were taught to distrust men. I wasn't quite sure why, but I did distrust them. The dogs would bark and my grandmother would nod. They do not like men. She would hold the collar of the angry dog as it jumped and snapped at the screen door when the man came to read the gas meter.

"I can't do anything," she would shrug. "She is unused to men."

I did well at school but there was almost always someone better.

"Did you get the top mark?" my grandmother would say when she knew I had a test.

"Second."

"Second is not good enough. You must be top. Next time you will be top."

I was an honest girl. I never lied, but I began to learn how to dodge her questions.

"Top of the class?"

"I'm not very good at this subject. I was only average," I would tell her, even if I had scored better than everyone else. She was disappointed, but soon the pattern of my invented failures became apparent.

"But you are good at art," she would say. "You are the best at sculpture. You are a sculptor. This is what you will be, the top sculptor."

My grandmother looms large in my memory, but we were a close-knit crew and my mother hugged me. I remember the pleasure of her lap, warm and comforting, and sometimes her hugs were harder than they should be. Sometimes they were for her own comfort and not for mine. I struggled free of her grasp and felt guilty when she seemed so lost and lonely. Once she told me that she would run away if she could, but I wasn't sure why. I was happy in the safe little nest and I knew nothing of the world beyond the boundaries of our garden.

I learned about sex in the schoolyard. I learned that it was something to do with whatever a man had in his pants and that special place in my body where the colors lived. I learned that this kind of thing made babies happen. I tried to imagine the shape of this man-thing, but I couldn't.

My grandmother and aunt were making a jazz band, a miniature orchestra of players each with a different instrument. My grandmother was tailoring clothes for them, vests and suit pants and pork-pie hats. I saw my grandmother pull the trousers out from one of the figures and peer inside them. She showed it to my aunt and they giggled together like girls in the playground giggle. I had never seen them behave like this before. I wanted to sneak up and pull the trumpet player's pants down and see how a man was made but when I tried, she had glued the waistband of his trousers to his hips. I couldn't even feel anything hidden when I pressed my fingers into the papier-mâché crotch.

THIS THING WITH PAUL

Brisbane 2008

Night. Sleepless night. A slight chill in the air, but I rest my hands under my laptop. The battery is a little fire to warm my fingers. Seven tabs open on the top of my screen. I flick from one to another, skimming. My husband is away, and without him there will be little sleep. His breath on my back is like chloroform; his absence is like coffee before bed. When I hear the little popping sound of a message coming through I am jittery.

Hello? Do you remember me?

I glance at the little pop-out box at the bottom of my Facebook page. Paul. A friend of Christopher's? I met him once at a writers' festival dinner.

I didn't know there was a chat function in Facebook.

Ah. Well there is.

The popping sound it makes is disconcerting.

Would you like me to stop talking to you?

No, actually, I am very happy to talk to you. I am having trouble sleeping.

I chat to Paul for an hour. We talk about writers and books and art. He seems to know a lot about things I am interested in. I try to remember his face and have a vague impression of someone short and perhaps a little brash; I can't picture him exactly.

I sit up in bed. I am beginning to enjoy the banter. When the battery is low I move to the lounge room where I can plug in. I am so far away from sleep by now. When Paul says he should go to bed I feel vaguely disappointed.

This is how it begins, unexpectedly. This Paul is now someone I know from the Internet more than real life; I didn't really take much notice of him at that dinner. I was distracted by a writer whose book I had quite enjoyed.

The next night, unsettled in my lonely bed, I look out for him, switching between Internet pornography and Facebook, where I will be able to see if he has come online. I am disappointed that he does not. I chat with someone else briefly, and without the same kind of connection. I find that I miss him; that I was looking forward to another conversation.

Strange how I hook into this thing with him so quickly. I turn over our conversation of the night before and his voice in my head sounds like my voice. Already, right up front, he feels like family to me.

BESTIAL

Blacktown 1978

There was a period I remember when I thought I would give birth to a creature that was half-dog, half-human. I dreamed it in those dark moments before wakefulness when reality is a meniscus of light at the very top of a deep well. I dreamed the thing was pink, squirmy, baby color, but with a fine coating of fur and black eyes and a long penis stretching the length of its belly and ending in a bright red worm that retracted its head when the creature breathed. In the dream I held the thing at arm's length, the hideous proof of what I had done.

What had I done? I sift back through the wrack of memory to find the moment.

Here is a small child at the top of the back stairs. It is hot and she—I; it is my memory after all—I have come here because this place is one of the few safe places in the whole of the house and garden. This tiny corner of the world makes me invisible. My mother, standing at the sink, can strain and stand on tiptoe but she will never see more than my shoes and only then if I choose to stretch my legs down to the second step.

It is hot and the dog is panting. It is a young dog, new to my house and more quick to play than the skittish saluki or the tetchy sheepdog or our labrador, who sleeps on my bed and presses her nose into my lap when I am crying.

Because of the extraordinary heat the new dog is calm for once. He is perched with his haunches pressed into my hip. I stroke his sleek fur, short and clean and gingerish. On this day he cannot settle. He sits and pants, shifting, stands and pants. I watch him, remembering all the times I have felt this way, itchy with heat, distracted by potential games but lacking the energy to chase them. I pat the inside of the dog's thigh, lean but meaty, like something that could be torn from a corpse and gnawed on. I am always thinking this kind of thing, although I know that I should not be. In a Dr. Seuss story I learned that I should only think of fluffy things or else I might just "thunk up a glunk." I simultaneously want, and also do not want, to thunk up a glunk.

The dog stands and shifts and his meat-bone thigh is at little-girl height and his penis is right here, panting in time to his breaths. The little red worm of it is slipping in and out of its velvety sheath.

I watch it.

Glunk, I think, don't thunk a glunk.

At school yesterday someone made a joke about moms and dads sleeping in the same bed and wearing no pajamas. Everyone laughed. I didn't.

"My mom and dad never slept in the same bed," I said, although I didn't really remember my dad sleeping in the same house as us at all.

"But they must have at some time."

"No."

"At least once."

"No."

And then the joke turned nasty, the little nip of giggles directed straight at me. Kiddie mirth like piranhas, I knew that this must be like the Santa Claus thing and that they would ultimately prove they were right and I was wrong.

The act, apparently, involved a dad putting his thing in and then some kind of white stuff and then a baby.

Here, on this hot concrete step, I look over at the new dog and its wormy thing and there is indeed some white stuff, just like they said there would be.

I am in this spot where no one can possibly observe me. If I were sitting anywhere else I would never do it but I am here, and so I will.

I touch it, the thing, and when I touch it, a drop of milk oozes onto my finger and I pull aside my knickers quickly and make it go where the kids at school have told me it should go.

The idea of a baby, half-dog, half-child, began to gestate in my imagination. There were weeks of secret nightmare births, of being followed by wolf-howls and padding shadows. I opened my legs in front of a mirror, checking for any signs of a bestial pregnancy, thinking that one day I might reach inside myself and feel the embryonic row of canines growing in a soft-furred skull.

I look back into the pit of my childhood and it is all sex and terror and art. I played branding and handball and I could throw and catch like a boy, but I was not a boy. I was not to play with the boys. I was coddled in the safe haven of my grandmother's house on Duckmallois Avenue, where men were wolves and strangers were to be treated like witches. Smile at them, nod, and then back quickly away.

My grandfather sat in the dark and listened to music on old 78s. Bach mostly, but some Beethoven, Puccini. Sometimes the music rose too loud and sharp to be borne without flinching. It was dynamic. There was a whole vast landscape inside it, stepped out by the runs of notes and cavernous silences. He let me sit in his favorite chair. It was a hard red globe and it spun when you kicked your feet against the floor. I sat and listened to his music even though I liked other music better. David Bowie, Kate Bush, *Dark Side of the Moon*, which my aunt listened to with her head resting on a pillow between the speakers. When she sat like that her bottom was left high and exposed to my grandmother's passing slaps and pinches.

Still, there was something subversive about my grandfather's music. The rest of my family hated his classical recordings. He was forced to play them in his room and preferred to do so in the dark. When my grandmother trotted past the door we heard her muttering complaints about the noise—"like a funeral"—and we grinned together without speaking.

He stuffed a pipe with tobacco and lit it, puffing hard to make embers glow. The smell of Dr. Pat was a pleasant one, rich and dark like the music. When the record came to the end of its groove he let me lift the needle, flip the heavy Bakelite, turn it. When I was younger still, he would supervise the turning of the record, holding the arm of the needle with me in case I dropped it, hovering nearby to catch the record if it slipped through my fingers. I turned fourteen, and I could be trusted as the rest of the family would not trust me.

His room smelled of chemicals, sharp and bitter. Behind us in the dark there were tables and benches and rows of synthetic rope strung across the corner from which to hang the drying prints. When he drew the curtains and pressed the Velcro down we succumbed to impenetrable blackness. He kept the black shades parted when we listened to music and when I raised my fingertips I could see them wriggling in the gloom.

Sometimes when he was at work I would sneak into his room, touch the covers of his records and hear the music resonating in my skull. In the dark, I would shuffle under the table where he developed his photographs and masturbate to the sound of Bach, the shut-up secretive smell of his den in my nostrils. Once he came home before I had finished. He knew I was there, my hand hidden under my skirt, but he pretended that he didn't. He shuffled some papers, lit his pipe, and then retreated, leaving me to finish in peace. I wondered if this was what he did here, too. I felt a kind of camaraderie with him because I knew that he must long for some kind of physical contact. He slept in a separate room, leaving my aunt and my grandmother their chaste twin beds.

Duckmallois Avenue was a reasonably pretty street, trying to hold its head up in a downtrodden area with a terrible reputation. Duckmallois Avenue turned its weatherboard back on rapes and murders, hung pretty floral blinds to shutter out the more insidious misdemeanors occurring in the neighbors' bedrooms. The lawns were tightly cropped inside picket fences, knee high and glistening with fresh paint. In some gardens there were roses, in others there were pretty annuals planted, tended, uprooted, replaced by seasonal bulbs and winter blooms. There was a German woman with an eye for garden ornaments, and a Greek family with pretty daughters, and older residents; no renters, no harried huddles of housing commission residences.

There were children, too, young boys who cruised slowly past on BMX bikes, stopping outside the heavy tangle of shrubs that made our house like no other on the street. Sometimes they slipped off the seats of their bicycles and crouched low to peer into the gloom. I knew that they were trying to catch a glimpse of us. Sometimes they threw stones that could not penetrate the thorny tangle. Sometimes they called out names. They thought that my grandmother was a witch, or perhaps that we were some kind of religious order. They had seen the two young girls, my sister and me, hurried from the car and into the house. They knew that we were not allowed to play on the street or in the little park just around the corner. They knew that we were a crowd of women, and if they had seen my grandfather skulking in the garden at twilight they did not mention it. Their curses were always female: witches, whores, harpies, sluts.

Inside our garden it was cooler than out there in the world. It was always dark and damp and there were special places; the branches low enough to climb on, the patches of tender leaves and the little purple violets that smelled sweet as clouds when you pressed your cheek into the leaf litter and breathed in hard.

I was not allowed out except for when I was walked to school by my mother or when we all went out together to the shops or to the movies. Sometimes they let me walk our pet ferret on a lead, but I was always accompanied by one of the adults. There were frequent family visits to the library and rare treats, journeys to the museum or the gallery. It was a goal of sorts, but I was not bothered beyond a slight sense of regret when other kids gathered for parties or school camp or when they talked about sleepovers, staying up all night playing games. I sensed instinctively that I would be out of place at the parties or sleepovers anyway. On camps I might spend my time alone. I read constantly, and when I was not reading or sneaking off to indulge myself in the pleasures of my newly swelling flesh, I helped the adults with their work or played games with my sister, arguing till mealtime.

My sister was three years older than me and she had just discovered Ayn Rand. Fat American novels that helped her to bully her way into a life of self-interest and capitalism. I had become obsessed by the Russian revolution, perhaps as a direct reaction to her change of style. I changed the pecking order on the chessboard, refusing to play unless the object was to protect every last pawn, killing off the aristocracy one by one. My sister called me Commie and Pinko. There was a cold war brewing in the darkest places of our garden fortress and I suspected that her armory was better stocked than mine.

FALLING IN LOVE
WITH YOUR FRIENDS

Brisbane 2008

I watch Christopher work and I am overwhelmed by my affection for him. He is tall and gentle-faced and when he bends to child-height there is nothing but affection as he takes the book out of the toddler's hand and waits patiently for the release of coins from his sweaty palms.

It is impossible to separate the urgency of this feeling from the urgency that fills me in the moments before an orgasm. It is all liquid pleasure and, dare I say it, love. I might be in love. I might be falling in love. I have somehow overstepped my vow of friendship and fallen into a place where my hard shell has dissolved. I am all soft-bodied mollusc. I am oyster and in this moment I would lay myself in his palm to be swallowed whole.

This is a pattern that I recognize. There is always someone

who can charm me out of my brittle protection, always a friend for whom I have unconditional love.

Just one friend at any one time, a kind of monogamous extramarital obsession. There is no language for me to explain the way I feel for Christopher as he wraps the book in a paper bag and passes it to the boy, solemn, respectful. I fall in love a little bit even though I said I wouldn't do that anymore. I can't help noticing his quiet dignity, his kindness. His subtle humor and, forced to stand so close in such a cramped workspace, there is the flesh as well, constantly brushing against mine. I try to love without lust but there is always lust. So, lust then, and a great heaped serving of love. Now there is this melancholy brew for me to drink down, slowly, on a day drawn out.

I am certain that this is only a fleeting wave of lust and soon, in a matter of days or weeks or months, I will transfer this affection to someone new. I am reminded of my conversation with Paul the other night on the Internet, the sudden intimacy, the wave of familial love, and something else, some unnameable emotion.

Sex addiction. Katherine was right. This is all about sex, because on top of the lust there is still the love I feel and will feel for him that will go on, even when this unwanted desire has moved off and onto someone new.

"You have to stop falling in love with your friends," my husband tells me. He has been watching me hop from one obsession to another for the eighteen years of our relationship.

"If I am a tap, and you are a sink," I tell him, "it is like I am locked on. A full-force gush of emotion and you are filled up with it, but there is too much. It is spilling out onto the floor. It is like I need to hold one bucket after another under the overflow. When the bucket is full I exchange it with another bucket."

I am pleased with my metaphor but he just shakes his head. "Well, you should stop falling in love with your friends. You'll chase them away," he tells me, voice of reason that he has always been.

"I am not monogamous and I am not heterosexual," I told my husband on the night we met.

I was sitting in a girl's lap. I liked her well enough. I had slept with her before in that easy way I used to enjoy. I would have slept with her again that night if I hadn't noticed Anthony. He was sitting on the floor, leaning against a wall. His deep green sweater was the exact color of the ocean at dusk. I noticed how blue his eyes were. His long hair pulled back and tied in a ponytail, the chiseled perfection of his cheeks.

I stopped kissing the girl. I switched from vodka to water. There was another drug present in the room and I felt myself turn toward it. I basked in the glow of potential sex. I hopped from one group to another, chatting briefly, moving ever closer to my target. Anthony was alone. He sat with a beer warming between his fists and smiled quietly, watching the crowd grow drunk and bleary-eyed.

He was beautiful. I had never before seen anyone quite as beautiful. I sat beside him quickly, before I could change my mind, and clicked my glass against his beer bottle as if we were old friends. I breathed through the erratic thudding of my heart, the exquisite tumble-turns low in my belly. I caught a whiff of his aftershave and a hint of soap. We talked about mutual friends, films, documentaries we had both enjoyed. We talked until we were amongst the last to leave. Maybe I would stay, sleep in a corner on the floor. Maybe he would stay, too, or maybe he would leave. Yes, I should leave. I said that I would walk home and so he offered me a lift.

"I am not heterosexual or monogamous," I told him, the sun climbing up over the silhouette of the city.

"You will be both of those things when you are with me." His prediction. And up until now I have proved him right with the slow torture of my abstinence, squirming with the fleeting possibility of other entanglements, struggling to contain the force of my love for one friend after another.

At the end of Christopher's shift we say goodbye and barely glance at each other. My heart breaks just a little for the string of people I have lusted after in this slow, sad way, love danced in time to the monotonous beat of the daily grind. Everything in its right place, except this little fragment of misplaced emotion that I have picked up like lint and curled into my hand with no place to rest it.

THE FIRST CENSORSHIP

Blacktown 1981

My sister gave me a book by Marion Zimmer Bradley for my birthday. It was set on a distant world, in a place far, far away, just like in a fairytale. I liked her books very much; I had been wanting to read this one for months. It would complete my collection, the collected works of Marion Zimmer Bradley.

There was a cake my grandmother had made and a little Princess Leia figure on top of it, her white robe sinking into the icing. There were thirteen candles, one of which had been placed too close to the action figure, and I watched as her face began to blister and blacken. My mother smothered the plastic girl in white icing and I washed her and vowed to love her more because of her disfigurement.

· I opened my presents and they were mostly books that I had coveted. I would read them all, but first I would read the book my sister gave me because I had been longing for the final Marion Zimmer Bradley for so long.

Someone had cut some of the pages out.

My mother saw me notice them and was quick to explain. "Just one bit that is adults only."

I counted the numbers on the bottom of the pages. I could feel my rage percolating inside me. There was the biley hiss of it just below the boil.

"It doesn't affect the flow of the story. There was just no need for that sex stuff."

That sex stuff.

I noticed the tight-lipped anger of my sister. This was her present to me and it had been hacked into, desecrated by the censors. I thought of all the books my sister had stolen from the library and passed to me in the dead of night. Banned books, books with love, kissing; sometimes more. I thought about the note I had to take to my English teacher excusing me from reading the set text because of the unsuitable content, and how my sister passed me an illicit copy of *1984* that I read using a flashlight under the covers late at night. An odd parallel between Orwell's world and my own.

We weren't allowed to visit any of our friends at their houses. We weren't allowed to get mail without my mother reading it. My mother was protecting us, I knew this. But I wasn't sure exactly what from.

I read that book late into the night. When I came to the missing pages I closed the book and imagined things that I had never seen written even in the banned books snuck to me by my sister after dark. I knitted in all the darkest possibilities, casting a spell to bind together the empty fragments of the missing pages. I thought about the worst things possible, the rapes and the ravaging, the fondling of the dead and the dying. I didn't flinch from any possibility in my imagination. I closed my eyes and pulled the covers over my head and I let myself stray into all the forbidden places that were unavailable to me in the sunlight world of my family's fairytale.

THE FIRST PORNOGRAPHY

It was hot the day of the school swimming carnival, a languid summer day smelling slightly acidic like the juice of an ant squashed between your fingertips, and I was signed up for the 200 meters.

I have always loved to swim. I swim very slowly but I can swim for hours at a time without tiring. I love the breathy rhythm of it, the way the surface of the water creeps above your ears, obliterating the world.

There were whispers about the photograph before anyone had seen it. Apparently the red-haired boy had it in his bag, a photograph of a woman with a carrot in her vagina. I lay on a towel in the sun and thought about how it would be to put a carrot in my vagina. I thought about the candles I sometimes smuggled into my bedroom and used late at night. I knew a carrot would be essentially the same, but somehow the idea of a vegetable inserted into someone's vagina played on my mind.

I thought that if there was a photo, there would have to have been a photographer. Someone watching the woman insert the carrot into her vagina. I wondered if she had gone into the next room, like an artist's model, and emerged with the carrot inserted, removing the light cotton sheet from around her shoulders, then lying or sitting on the divan with the carrot neatly in place.

My race was next. I had never been in a race before. I had never worn my swimsuit in front of my peers. I wondered suddenly if I should have signed up for the race at all. I still had the usual exemption note from my mother; would it be too late now to table it and have myself scratched?

I was wondering this when someone brought me the photograph. Not a real photograph but a picture of one, torn from a magazine. Sepia. Old. It reminded me of the elegantly posed portraits of our great-grandmothers, only this grandmother was not wearing any clothes and there was a carrot in her vagina.

I needed to take my school dress off. I was wearing my bathing suit underneath. Everybody else had already changed into their suits and lay in the lazy spread of the hot bleachers or flat on their backs with their knees spread to make an even tan.

I could never lie like that.

I folded the photograph into the novel that I had been reading, even though Wendy Jones was waiting to see it, and stashed it deep inside my schoolbag.

I pulled the sack of check fabric over my head. The corner of it snagged on my glasses. New ones, pink government-issue glasses with little upward curls at each edge. In a few days I would lose them as I always did and it would be six months before I could get a new pair. I wondered when my mother would tire of replacing them. I folded them roughly and shoved them in beside my novel.

I stood at the starting block. The other girls wore bikinis and had sleek flat chests and skinny hips. I was too round. I was aware of my new breasts, which were already so large that you could hold a pencil under them. I had read about this in someone's magazine. Are my breasts too floppy? Answering the multiple-choice questions when no one was looking.

I missed the starting gun but I plummeted anyway, a moment's delay and then the fat slap of water, the bliss of submerged oblivion.

I thought about the woman with the carrot in her vagina. Did the cameraman adjust the carrot, moving it a little this way or that, pushing or pulling? I wondered how these things could be orchestrated. I wondered if the woman had family, if she told her mother about the photographer, if she married him or perhaps had children with him. I wondered if the photographer might have been a woman. Would it be easier to have a woman moving your carrot a little farther in, a little farther out? I wondered about the hundreds of people who had seen this photograph since then. I thought about that woman with the carrot and her ability to bring a whole new generation of teenagers to orgasm.

I saw the blue-tiled wall approaching. Half the race over. I kicked and my arms windmilled and I reached out for the tiles, felt them beneath my fingers, was about to turn and head for the finish line when I felt a hand on my shoulder.

I bobbed to the surface, panting. One of the teachers was leaning into the pool and tapping my head. There was a waterfall of hair in my eyes but I could see that there were no other swimmers in the pool. The others had finished their race. I was only halfway through.

"I can finish," I gasped. It was only another fifty meters.

"They're waiting to start the next race. You can get out at this end now. Better not hold the races up."

I nodded, ducked under the little colored floaties marking the lanes. I emerged from the pool in my one-piece swimsuit and everyone was watching me. I knew that I should be embarrassed, but I wasn't. I sat with my towel and my schoolbag beside me and the photo of the woman with a carrot that I would sneak home and stash under my bed. I had just procured my first piece of pornography. There would be many more.

COUNSELED

Brisbane 2008

"I think I have a sexual addiction."

She sits in a chair a long way away from mine. She has a pleasant face. I like her immediately. She seems intelligent, human. I can see myself being honest with her. I want to be honest. I am paying a lot of money to be honest with her.

"Why is it you think that? How is this addiction expressed?"

We have an hour together. I wonder how it is possible to even scratch the surface of it in an hour. How to explain that I have built my life around sex; I think about it almost every waking moment.

"I masturbate all the time," I tell her, "I can't survive a day without it." I tell her how it eats into my time. When I am at home, struggling with my writing, I trawl for pornography on the Internet. I download free grabs, quick little shots of the stuff, consumed like amyl nitrate. The rush is instant and relieving. Once or twice I have been caught out by the postman or someone visiting, once at work I was discovered indulging in my fix in the upstairs office when I had arrived an hour early for my shift. None of this really bothers me. I have never let the sex distract me from my job; apart from a little awkwardness if I am ever interrupted, it is a relatively benign habit.

"And then I sexualize everybody. I think about sleeping with them. There's this thing I do where I pick someone as my friend and then I fall in love with them." To date, however, I have not acted on any of these desires. They are all unrequited longings, fuel for the furtive moments of procrastination. If anything they only serve to augment the ever-satisfying marital bed. They are little forays into the unknown from which I slip back into the real world with small gems that I have picked up from my imaginary lovers. Sometimes I surprise my husband with my inventiveness. Eighteen years of marriage and the palette has only become richer.

"Yes," she says. "What about your husband?"

My beautiful boy. My first impulse is to speak about my lust. The thought of him precipitates a surge in my groin. I can feel the drug of my desire shooting out into my brain, spreading its anemone fingers down into my spine. But it is more than lust.

"He is family," I tell her. "Familial love."

I don't believe in romantic love, the neatness of the fairytale. I am certain the world is too chaotic to accommodate such an organized concept, but the idea of it is delicious. I want to tell her about Christopher, and the one before him, and the one that will be after. I want to impress her with my tap-and-bucket analogy. I want to tell her about my inability to separate my unconditional care from my lust, that ever-present engine that powers my body, keeping it on edge at the point of fight or flight. I want to tell her that even as I begin to feel this way, I am waiting for the moment when I will have no words and I will reach out to touch and be slapped back, laughed at, belittled.

"I think I have a problem with intimacy," I tell her; I see her glance at her watch. Almost time.

"A problem?"

That may in fact be an understatement.

"You have a problem with intimacy, but you say you have no problem with sex?"

"Oh no. No problem with sex. Sex is clean. Easy. Sex has nothing to do with intimacy."

She raises an eyebrow and I know the question already. I replay myself: sex has nothing to do with intimacy. I am certain that other people would disagree with me. She would disagree with me, but I know quite a bit about sex and I am certain that sex and intimacy are completely separate in the scheme of things.

I walk back to the shop where Christopher has an armful of books for shelving. Customers glance toward me and I wonder if my little disclosures are written on my skin. I notice how the rest of the staff are easy with each other. I notice how they give me space, careful not to brush by me, cautious, tiptoeing around me as if I were radioactive.

I am twice their age. I am the old woman of the bookstore. I wonder what they think of my constantly crude conversation, my continuous sexualization of the warm bodies walking through the door. I wonder if they laugh about me after work when they gather to watch bands or drink beer. I wonder if I have become a joke, the aging sexpot from the bad seventies television shows. I wonder when I first realized that sex and intimacy are entirely different things.

WINNING LOTTO

Blacktown 1982

On Wednesday evenings we watched the television. We never watched the news like the other kids at school. The news was "all wars and killing and hate." We were allowed to watch family-friendly sitcoms, *I Love Lucy* and *I Dream of Jeannie* and *Bewitched*, but the television would be turned off if Samantha kissed Darren for longer than her usual peck on the cheek. On Wednesday nights my grandmother put on her large-rimmed spectacles and settled with her calculator and her notepad and rows of complicated calculations.

"I do my maths," she said, the television flickering in the background, too low to hear the voices.

She had devised a formula. On one side of the page she played this out, line after line of long division, multiplication, equations, substituting numbers for the letters that took their place at the top of the page. My aunt double-checked her addition using a calculator, duplicating the set of numbers, cross-checking. This seemed to be the work of hours, and the rest of us, the other three, were left to talk or to sit in the lounge chairs reading our books. I glanced up, wondering if I would be missed if I disappeared to the bathroom for a while. I had to pick my moments; perhaps it was too soon after the last trip. I decided I could wait it out. Maybe after the lotto was over, when everyone was getting ready for dinner.

The woman on the television, too pretty to be beautiful, wore a big fake blond smile. The man had hair that might be molded plastic, too dark. The numbers fell, and the women ticked and clucked. When I was younger I had sacrificed my pocket money to the general lottery fund. From time to time there would be a win. I would have to choose between a brand new paperback from a proper, new bookshop or an animal, a pet of some kind. A string of doomed guinea pigs, rabbits, turtles, lizards, and fish ensued. I was determined. I continued to invest. But when Gruesome the ferret died, I decided the pleasure the animals brought did not justify the mourning period. I withdrew my financial support for the betting syndicate and saved my dollars, buying my own paperbacks at the secondhand bookshop whenever I had accrued enough.

On this night I had no investment in the fall of the numbers. I glanced up now and then as my grandmother and aunt crowded around their little notebook. They were whispering, checking, flipping back and forth between pages, underlining their calculations. Another win, I suspected. Every week it seemed there was at least one game that came in a winner, twenty dollars here, fifty dollars there. They would earn their fortune one crisp new note at a time, except that they always invested more than was returned.

When we win the lotto, they said, we will take holidays to Broadbeach every week. We will buy pretty dresses for you girls, new slacks for us. We will buy that crocodile skeleton in the shell shop at The Rocks. We will buy you the complete set of Ray Bradbury stories. We will move away from Blacktown and we'll build a dream world, Xanadu, just like in the poem. A stately pleasure dome, caverns measureless to man, like Disneyland, only better. Much better than Disneyland because the papier-mâché models that we make are nicer. Roller coasters, haunted houses, a mirror maze, a gingerbread house, a forest of flowers big as trees, a forest of trees as small as flowers. There will be a little train running through it and all the children can sit on top of it and chug along through our wonderland.

My grandmother watched *Willy Wonka and the Chocolate Factory* over and over on video. She called it Willy Wanker, and after my sister and I had exhausted our snickering over her mispronunciation, we would sit with her, watching as she paused the video, standing up close and leaning over the hulking screen of the old TV, pointing. A chocolate river, like that, only we could have lily pads for stepping-stones. We could put giant chocolate frogs, not chocolate, really, papier-mâché, but made to look like chocolate. What you think Sheila? When the lotto numbers fall for us—yes? And my aunt would nod, seriously considering the technicalities of this confectionous feat of engineering.

But on this night there was a win, I was certain of it. There was a little electric thrill of excitement as they checked and double-checked the numbers. Even my mother had lifted herself out of her chair to join them. A win, definitely, and not just a twenty-dollar win. Maybe as much as five hundred dollars and perhaps we would put on our best clothes and get on the train and spend Sunday at The Rocks, picking through shelves of Sepik art, fossils buried in stone. If we had a win then there might be scones with jam and cream in some little backstreet courtyard café.

"Did you win?"

My aunt was quick to answer. "Not really." Too quick.

"We have to check it. A little win maybe." I knew my grandmother was lying. When they had a little win she would stand up and cheer. She would gloat about the system she had developed, crank the handle on their little toy lotto wheel and let the balls fall into a neat row where she could count them. She would sit with my aunt for an hour after the lotto draw congratulating herself on her mathematical prowess, or, if there was no little win, she would check back through pages of calculations to see where they went wrong, adjusting their formula to make their chances of winning more solid.

On this night they closed their lotto journal immediately. They sat in silence. My aunt inserted a cigarette into a spidery black cigarette holder as long as my hand and lit it. My grandmother lit her own smoke off her daughter's and stuffed it into a shorter holder. My mother shook her lighter and found sparks three times before there was a flame. She puffed and I breathed in the sweet minty odor of her smoke.

My mother couldn't settle that night. She creaked back and forth in her lounge chair. My aunt and grandmother were surprisingly still, staring at the blank face of the television. I was not used to seeing my grandmother sit still for so long. It made me slightly nervous.

"There is a little bit of crème de menthe," my mother said, "left over from Christmas."

Crème de menthe. It wasn't anyone's birthday. It wasn't Easter, they hadn't just completed one of their displays for a council library. It was an ordinary weeknight and they were talking about crème de menthe.

"Wendy! Please!" My grandmother chided as if she had suggested we all take off our clothes and run naked down Duckmallois Avenue.

"Just a little glass."

My grandmother held up a stern finger. "If you feel like it still, tomorrow night, after—" she left space for an unspoken fragment of her sentence. The others nodded.

I looked toward my sister. She was still scowling into her copy of

The Fountainhead. She had heard the exchange but, unlike me, refused to be curious. Their business had nothing to do with her. She was an island separated from us by the bristling of her back.

"All right," my mother conceded. "Tomorrow night."

My grandmother warned, "It might be something wrong. A mistake."

"Ah! Ah! Ah!" My aunt glanced toward my sister and me, both of us pretending to be engrossed in our novels.

"I'm not saying," my grandmother said. "I just mean not to count your eggs."

"Chickens," my aunt corrected her.

Chickens, eggs, crème de menthe. This is how I came to realize that the win was not a little one at all. First-division lotto, which meant there was no trip to the rocks to buy Sepik art. There were no scones with strawberry jam. Instead there was a promise of something entirely more grand.

"We are going to move to Dragonhall," they told me. "But it is a secret. Don't tell them at school. If they know you are leaving they might stop caring about you in class. They might fail you because they are jealous. Don't tell your teachers until we are all packed and ready to get on the plane."

"Where is Dragonhall?" I asked them.

They pointed to the map, somewhere in Queensland, a place

near the ocean, a fly-spot labeled Bororen with the blue of the sea less than a finger reach away.

"This is our Disneyland," my grandmother told me. "Dragonhall because my name, Dragitsa, means dragon."

"No," Sheila corrected. "It means Charlotte, Lotty. A female version of Charles."

"Yes, Charlie; but it is also like a dragon, my family's symbol had a dragon."

"A dragon on the top of it," my aunt confirmed.

"Dragon-hall. You want to go to Dragonhall?"

Of course I wanted to go to Dragonhall. I wanted to go away from a school where I was harassed by older kids and abandoned by my sister. I wanted to stop being afraid that the man who raped a neighbor and carved his initials in her skin might climb in through my bedroom window and carve his name in me. I wanted to live in a place that was like Disneyland only better.

I went to bed early and slept without the nightmares that always plagued me. Instead I dreamed of chocolate frogs, gingerbread forests, and measureless caverns dripping with stalactites. The promise of Dragonhall.

THIS THING WITH PAUL 2

Brisbane 2008

Paul is there again. Most people put their own image on their Facebook page but he has a piece of art. A house, balanced on a mountainous peak, a wash of a storm brewing. I have come to associate the picture that stands in for him with pleasure. I smile when I see it and when I am anxious I close my eyes and there is his house behind them like a reassurance. I know it is silly, but I associate our chats with a feeling of contentment and his picture is enough to evoke this feeling. He chats to me about books and styles of writing.

I have started a blog, I tell him, because I am jealous of Christopher's "Furious Horses," writing a new story every day.

What is it called?

"Furious Vaginas."

Hahaha, he says and then it seems he is gone. A silence which I punctuate with question marks at intervals.

I like that it isn't about sex. He is back again.

Isn't it?

No, he says. It seems to be about other things.

I ask him to send me some of his work. I have heard that his writing is good but I am not sure that I have read any of it. We talk about Nicholson Baker as he gathers things together to send as a file. Paul multitasks like a demon. This, more than anything, marks him as a member of the next generation. I know that I am far too old for him. I am from a different era.

Vox is about us, I say. You and me.

Ah, but I never talk about sex.

But I do.

Therefore *Vox* is about you, but not about us, exactly.

You will talk about sex one day, I tell him. I will have an influence on you.

When you talk about sex, Paul says, you are not actually talking about sex.

And so of course I answer, When you talk about other things you are always talking about sex but in an oblique way.

And then the file comes down. I click over to my Gmail and they are there, Paul's stories. A little paperclip and beneath it three small files. I open them. A new message from Paul makes a little popping sound, but I ignore it. He will know I am reading. His stories are good, clever. One of them is funny and it makes me smile. It is not until I open the third one that I feel my heart engaging. This story goes on too long. There is a moment when I feel my chest expanding, my heart opening up to him, my eyes pricking with tears, and then the story moves on a little, like a train that has overshot the station, leaving the passengers stranded with no platform to step down onto. I switch to chat and tell him this and he immediately starts to fix the thing. He sends me an amendment, which seems better.

I can't believe you went and changed it just like that.

Why wouldn't I if it makes it better?

I don't know, because you are a young person. Young people are precious about their work.

I like to edit, he tells me. I like to make things better.

I like you, is my reply. I like you very much. I like your stories. If you ever write a novel I might develop a crush on you.

I am not sure I will write a novel. I may be a short story writer. I like short stories.

Ah well, then you will never have my unwanted romantic attentions.

This is a risk I will have to take, Paul tells me, and I laugh. He makes me smile and he makes me laugh.

When Paul signs off for the night I go back into his Facebook page just to look at the little house perched precariously in the storm.

It is a beautiful image, painted by a friend of his. I like the painting on its own merits but I also now associate it with our conversations. Looking at it, I feel a liquid rush. I become unsettled. I know that I'll have to masturbate or I will never sleep.

Oh, so now I have become sexually attracted to an image that stands in for a person that I can only vaguely remember in real life. The physical representation of Paul is that image. I lie on the couch and watch it as I place my hand quietly between my legs, and the release is quick and violent. When it is done there is still the picture on the screen and I really can't remember what he looks like in real life. When I close my eyes there is a little house on a hill and I must not concentrate on it too closely because I can already feel the warmth of desire rising up in me for a second time, and if I give in to this I will never get to bed.

My boy is sleeping on his side and the light on his face is a real and beautiful thing. Strange to be able to masturbate over someone else's profile picture and not feel my love and desire for my husband at all diminished.

I know better than to wake him with my caresses at this point. He will be tired and irritable. I lie beside him and I am wide awake and he smells like hot dough, baking, and I want to take him into my mouth. My desire for it is difficult to ignore. As I wonder vaguely if I should get up and release the pent-up energy discreetly in the lounge room, I find that I am yawning. I turn over onto my side and leap desperately for a wave of sleep.

MOVING ON
Blacktown 1983

Something crashed outside. There were muffled voices. The kitchen was being packed away. The ancient boxes of jelly and custard with their out-of-date faces grinning on the packets, the tins so old they had lost their labels, the more recent purchases of tomatoes, beans, rice. All of this was being transferred to boxes. We would ferret around in these, piecing together our makeshift meals while the kitchen was being painted. The house was a mess of boxes and baskets. There was always someone running one way or the other. We were moving to Dragonhall and although we were exhausted by the weight of packing there was a playful joy in the air.

My grandfather was separate from this activity. He was responsible for his own room. There were boxes leaning up against the cupboard but he had made no effort to assemble them. His enlarger still crouched in its corner, the trays for developer and fixative were still laid out side by side.

The night before we left I listened to Bach with him, squinting through the dark to catch some glimmer of change, but he was impassive. I wondered if anyone had even told him that we were moving. He had taken to eating his meals in his room in the dark, with the music turned up loud enough to obliterate any trace of the women of the house. He listened to the news in the morning and again at midday and before dinner. He shuffled out, stiff with too much sitting, to shower and shave and sometimes he wandered into the forest of our front yard to stand with the hose turned on the ferns and the river oaks and the pots of herbs bordering the porch.

He had separated himself from the others. When they spoke to each other it was to convey some practical information: "Do you want porridge or toast for breakfast?" "We are all going down to the shops, lock the door if you go outside." "Please can you turn that racket down, I can't even think with your violins blazing." If they had spoken to him about the move to Queensland, then it was when I wasn't in the house. I couldn't tell if he was as excited about the move as the rest of us. It seemed that he would grow roots, hunkering down when we were disentangling ourselves from Blacktown.

Nonetheless, we would be leaving. One bag for each person, carry-on luggage. Mine was mostly books and a few scant changes of clothing; my pajamas, which I was wearing now and would stuff into the bag when it was morning. The next time I wore them I would be there. There was still cleaning to be done and I helped as much as I could, but there was a point when tempers flared and the cleaning turned to bickering and the dogs, sensing that there was some major change encroaching, stayed in their corners whimpering. The great dane rose and paced and was shouted at and settled momentarily before rising again. I kissed them all goodnight, received an affectionate slap from my grandmother and squeezed past boxes, past places in the corridor where a younger version of myself saw phantom children scampering and the place where my sister held me down and tickled me till I urinated on the floorboards, and the far end of the corridor where our games of Minotaur would end with me crouched and weeping in the dark as my sister loomed over me and growled low in her throat like an angry wolf.

When I reached my aunt's study, where we would be sleeping amongst the boxes and the stacked furniture, I felt I had run the gauntlet. I was restless, ready to move forward into an adventure.

"If you tell them, I'll kill you."

I did not see my sister at first. She was hunkered down behind wrapped paintings, squeezed together with packaging tape. I could see the faint glow of blue light and when I stepped over piles of boxes to the mattress on the floor that we would be sharing, I realized that the television was there. She had peeled back the cardboard from the front and slung a blanket over it, tenting herself close up to the faint hum of the volume turned down low. It was against the rules to watch the TV unsupervised, particularly after dark when we might catch a glimpse of something scandalous.

"I'll let you watch if you promise not to tell your family."

She had taken to calling them that—your mother, your aunt—as if they were unrelated to her, extracting herself from their fierce familial hug.

When I crawled onto the mattress with her I felt my heart pounding. One glance at the screen and I was ready to brave the punishment alongside my sister because there, in the tantalizing veiled light, was David Bowie. This, then, must be the film that I had read about and never seen. *The Man Who Fell to Earth.*

"Have I missed much?"

"No. Just started."

We settled down together, unlikely conspirators given our checkered history. From what I had read this film would be much worse than PG, which was the only rating that we were allowed to watch. This was at least an R rating in its uncut form.

Bowie bounced naked and there was his penis. I had never seen a human penis before. This tiny wormy thing, this little piece of ropey flesh was what all the fuss was about. I was incredulous and yet aroused, mostly by the covert nature of the viewing. When the penis disappeared from the screen I longed to see it again. A penis in the flesh, not just the vague representations in art, little lumps of stone at the crux of sculptures, startling overstatements on the walls of Egyptian tombs. This was a human penis and it was like nothing I could have anticipated. It was way past my bedtime and I was glued to the screen. Drug use, violence, sex.

There was a sound in the corridor. We snapped the television off and listened, trembling under the covers, until we heard the toilet flushing and whoever it was walked back to the lounge room and shut the door. We giggled, sisters suddenly, and I wished I had been brave enough to do this before, join my sister on her adventures, break the rules and laugh and never once care that I might be caught.

I had my own secrets, of course. I hid objects in my bedroom that were long and thin enough to engage in sexual experimentation: candles, pencils, things with rubbery textures, costume jewelry, necklaces that could be inserted and removed stone by stone.

The only door that could be locked inside the house was the bathroom and so I would smuggle my toys in there hidden amongst my clothing. I was fond of long baths. I had a repertoire of lascivious images borrowed from the banned books and I took them out and turned them over in my memory until they were worn thin and smooth. I learned to hurry toward my silent orgasms. I practiced till I could come quickly and often, in the same way that other teenagers practiced smoking: hurried puffs, and all the evidence removed before anyone chanced by.

Here in the quiet moments, when the film had played out its

terrible conclusion, I was tempted to share my secret with my sister. I was obsessed by sex. I wanted to tell her I touched myself; a lot, several times a day. I wanted to ask my sister if she did the same, and if there was someone out there in the world that she thought about when she did it. I wanted to know if there was anyone she loved that she would be leaving behind.

But we had been assigned a double mattress on the floor and I was afraid that my confession would shatter the tenuous collegiality. I turned my back to her and said goodnight and waited to hear her fall asleep. Instead she sighed and tossed restlessly for a while before turning toward me.

"I don't want to go to Queensland," she said, less than a whisper, just breath and the shape of the words on her quiet lips. "I won't stay there for long."

I shifted onto my back, afraid to look at her in case she raised the barriers once more.

"I'm eighteen next year," she told me. "Hicksville, backwater, country bumpkins. I'll work for a year and then I'll take off."

"Where will you go?"

"Anywhere. Away."

She settled down with her back toward me and I was careful not to touch her skin under the blankets. In normal circumstances she would never share a bed with me but this was different. One more night and we would be gone.

I could smell the weedy scent of river oaks, chill air, the sound of my family working late into the morning, scrubbing cupboards and painting skirting boards. Occasionally there would be a little tinkle of laughter; sometimes a yelp as one dog or another was tripped over or stood on.

I could smell the constant stream of tobacco smoke, one cigarette after another. My sister's breath weighed heavy with sleep. The sunlight began to seep into the sky and I wasn't ready for a new day.

The movers would be arriving in a matter of hours. Perhaps they had already packed the pots and pans and I would have to face the day without a coffee.

I closed my eyes and tried to force myself to sleep, but I was held at arm's length from oblivion by a fluttering that was half my own excitement, half my sister's foreboding and when the door was flung open, "Krissy, Karen, better get up now," I was already too exhausted to lift my head.

HETEROSEXUAL
AND MONOGAMOUS

Brisbane 2008

I am folding my husband's clothes into vaguely neat piles when I remember the night we met. Strange how memory works, the scent of the washing powder, which hasn't dissolved completely and clings to the crotch of his jeans in little white clumps. I turn the sleeves over a shirt, trying to replicate Anthony's obsessive neatness, and I am transported to the chaos of my flat and the sight of a man crawling through the window.

He woke my husband, who was not my husband yet. I blinked at his beautiful face and couldn't, in fact, remember his name. I thought it might be Andrew but I was too shy to try it out in case I was mistaken.

The man was my neighbor but Andrew wasn't to know that. A short man, the neighbor, barely five foot two, round and with a lot of hair. You could see the hair poking out from the top of the towel wrapped around his waist. A shirt of hair clothing his entire upper body, and the hair on his head kept long, cascading down his back in a ponytail. My neighbor hefted himself up through the window and hit the floor with a thud, and my husband woke.

We both glanced up at the man climbing through my window with only a towel wrapped around his waist.

"Oh," he said, and, "sorry. I didn't realize . . ." and he left by the door, pulling it gently shut behind him.

"I have never slept with him," I told my husband. I measured people in this way at the time, dividing them up into lovers and ex-lovers, potential lovers and those I would not sleep with. Scant few. My neighbor included.

"Okay Kathy."

And I laughed. "I don't remember your name either."

"You will," he said.

It sounded like a line. "Ah. Will I."

"Yes. You won't be able to get rid of me."

I shuffled up to sitting, pulled the pillow comfortably behind my back.

"Andrew," I said.

"Anthony."

"Anthony, then. I am not heterosexual or monogamous."

He nodded. "I understand, but you will be while you are with me."

"And will I be with you?"

"Yes."

"Really? For how long?"

"Long enough."

He kissed me then, and it was nice. Kissing wasn't a thing I prided myself on, but there was a tenderness behind this kiss and I drank it down. I felt like coffee and a cigarette but a kiss would do. We were disturbed by the shudder of the window being opened again and another man, another neighbor, spidered his way over the sill.

"Oh," he said, but he tiptoed into the room regardless, reached for a guitar that was resting against a wall, nodded, waved and scrambled out through the window once more, all jangly strings and echoing wood.

"I've slept with him," I told my husband.

"Heterosexual and monogamous, Kathy."

"Krissy."

He kissed me. I liked it. I didn't believe him then, but now, eighteen years later, I wonder how he knew.

DRAGONHALL

Bororen 1983

I stood on the floor and looked out through the bones of the unfinished house. The walls would go up tomorrow but they had laid the floor first, which made no sense to me. It looked like a dance floor, polished wood running straight and shiny from one side of the house to the other, still open to the elements. I stood on the polished boards and imagined the tracks of kangaroos bouncing over the floorboards, brown snakes propelling their sinewy bodies over the slithery surface, cane toads, hundreds of them, congregating in what would become my bedroom.

It was like two houses conjoined. Our side of the house had three bedrooms, one each for my mother, my sister, and me. Their side of the house had three bedrooms, for my aunt, my grandfather, and my grandmother. There were two doors between the divided camps and we could lock them, separating into our natural divisions. In the middle, a shared space the size of a lounge room. No man's land. A room to be fought over, just like the place where my grandmother was born. There had always been a divide in the family, and here it had been drawn out, the differences between us made explicit by the pattern of the rooms.

Dragonhall itself would be on the adjacent property. My grandmother stepped us through it, walking through the jaws of the dragon into the entryway where you would pay your money, buy your gifts. Beyond this there were rooms set up with different tableaux. Fairytales in one part. Snow White, Sleeping Beauty, Rumpelstiltskin, Puck and the Fairy Mountain, the Little Match Girl. Then the real life. Dinosaurs, Egyptian mythology. They seemed to have abandoned the idea of the chocolate lake and the little train for children to ride from room to room. Scaled down, it still seemed that Dragonhall would be a proud monument to their years of work.

For the moment they had built a Besser Brick shed and all the models were stored in this. There were damages. My grandmother pulled Alice out of a box. Alice had appeared in libraries across the western suburbs, peering out from behind a giant mushroom at the riot of a tea party gone wrong. The plates upended, the guests asleep in coffee cups. A mother nursing a pig in a baby suit, a rabbit checking his watch. Now I saw how her fingers had been bent, the surface layer of plaster cracked, the paint chipped and peeling. I touched her damaged face, brushing aside the wave of sandy blond hair. Real human hair, from the head of a school friend of mine who had told me she was cutting her long blond ponytail off. (I had been distraught, pretty girls should never lose their hair. My own hair was a harsh and scratchy mat of dark curls and I stroked the softness of these locks and wished I could exchange my hair for hers.) I had told my family the story and my grandmother was ready with an offer for the soon-to-be-abandoned hair. Alice looked beautiful wearing my friend's hair tied back from her face by a blue band of silk.

Now I touched her shattered cheek and stroked her hair. I remembered the transaction, a scalp paid for in full, but I could barely remember my friend at all.

I walked through the grounds of the schoolyard, such a little place, a few portable classrooms, a permanent building, a little stretch of asphalt for the kids to play on. The school only held classes up to grade ten. I noticed the bored teenagers clustered around the park, sneaking cans of beer under their sweaters. They scowled at me distrustfully. New kid, city kid, fat kid. It reminded me of the kids at Blacktown, watchful creatures waiting for their opportunity to strike.

My mother told me that most of them just dropped out after grade ten. There were jobs on their parents' farms. Plenty of work to be done. I noticed the groups of older boys, their predatory glances as they leaned together on the balcony of the pub.

I sat in the middle of our yard and there was something settling over me that I couldn't shake, a sense of dread, a tight feeling in my chest, a howling loneliness like wind through a gutted building. We were all crammed into a little space and there was no time for privacy. There was always someone waiting for the bathroom. There was my sister on a twin mattress on the floor. There were dogs edging me out of my blankets. I had no space and no alone time and my body was edgy from lack of release.

My sister found me sitting amongst the dry grasses. She noticed the mood I was in, and I was surprised when she chose to sit beside me as if we were friends.

"What's up?"

"I don't know. I feel horrible."

"Sick?"

"Not exactly. It's like I'm empty and there's no way to fill it. I've never felt like this before. I can't make it stop and that's all I want. I want it to go away."

She seemed pleased by this. She settled closer.

"Finally," she said. "You're always like Pollyanna. Looking on the bright side of everything. But life's just not like that. There is no bright side. Everything is horrible and then we die. I'm proud of you for finally recognizing this."

I was confused. I was grateful that at last she approved of me. It made me feel more adult, like I'd shed my childish skin and crawled, pale as a new insect, into the world. Still I wanted to crawl back into the safe cocoon that had shielded me from this gnawing emptiness.

"If I died then at least I wouldn't feel like this anymore," I said.

She leaned over and hugged me. My sister never touched me; for a moment I'd thought she was going to hit me, but her arms were strong and comforting and I sank into them with relief. I let myself cry into her shoulder and she squeezed me so hard that some of my tears were from pain.

"Welcome to reality," she told me. "You've finally grown up."

The loneliness did not disappear, but my sister and I shared a tenuous friendship.

"Resign yourself," she said. "You will never be successful. Look at them." Them, the others, that lot: her way of referring to our family. "Look at them. Pathetic. Wanting to be successful. Happy. There is no such thing as happiness."

I looked at them, my family. The house was still being built. Dragonhall was still being built. Their dreams were still brimming with potential, but inside this hormonal sulk we shared I began to doubt the possibility of success.

We lay for hours on the front lawn of the rented house, my sister and I, side by side in our swimsuits, trying for a tan. My sister pinked up quickly, but I had inherited my grandfather's swarthy skin and my plump limbs turned to charcoal in the sunlight. A yellow truck rattled by and the back of it was filled with young men in tank tops and khaki work pants. My sister raised her roasting body up on her elbows and stared combatively straight at them. The truckload of workers broke into spontaneous cheering.

Under the darkness of my tan I could feel a blush sweeping across my skin. They were cheering for her, for us. I had never been looked at or whistled at by boys before. I was the fat weird girl who reads too much. I was the one they laughed at, never to be cheered for.

We waited for another truck to pass and when it did we both rose up to challenge it. Another cheer, and whistling this time; I felt as if the speed and the distance had disguised the hideous puffiness of my flesh. My sister held up her middle finger and this defiant gesture earned her an excited round of applause.

"I'm going to take my top off," I told her.

I knew she didn't believe me, but when the next truckload of workers passed I lowered the top of my one-piece swimsuit and the cheers were explosive.

We lay back, giggling and breathless.

"If you could see ten years into the future, who do you think you would be with? Would you have a boyfriend? A husband?"

She snorted, turned over onto her front to scald her back in the sun. "No. I think we'll both be sad and alone."

. . .

The yellow truck stopped. The nameless men vaulted over its railings, ran toward our garden. They were all tight arms and shining sinew. They were ripe with heat and strength and sweat and when they were close enough to cast a shadow over me I felt afraid. My legs were shaking. I wanted this. I pulled down my swimsuit and exposed my breasts to them. I had wanted them to stop for me, but now that they had I felt afraid. The fear was a shiver that vibrated the muscles under my skin. I crossed my legs coyly and the pressure of this movement created a wet warmth in my crotch.

In the dream they circled me and I felt their shadows dark and cold like sharks brushing against my legs. My fear silenced me. The first man to break this circling standoff was slick with sweat. He kneeled, straddling my crossed legs, and it was at the encouragement of the others that he slipped his hand between my legs and his finger, rough from work and smelling like soil, dragged the crotch of my swimsuit aside and I felt the scratch of it entering me. I was trembling by then and my fear was like excitement.

Hands on both my legs, hands around my wrists. Four men stretching me taught as a skinned roo and the fabric of my swimsuit gave way so easily when he wrenched it to one side. The heavy chest pushing the air from my lungs. The scent of sweat and hay and diesel, the tugging of the hands around my limbs. I was acutely aware of each of these sensations and if I woke before the first man had finished with me and zipped up, stepping aside for another man to take his place, then I would be disappointed. I would crush my fist between my legs and roll over hoping to regain the rising tide of excitement before the last fragments of sleep drifted away.

It was a recurring dream, and when it didn't recur of its own accord I sought it out. I made it happen again and again and again.

SCHOOL AGAIN

Somehow my mother had negotiated for me to hitch a ride with the special school bus that would pick me up from the Turkey Road turn-off and drop me at the Boyne Island stop. From there, the Gladstone bus would take me to school. We hauled ourselves into the consumptive Kombi and my mother bunny-hopped the hulking thing across the corrugations of the access road.

"If the bus doesn't connect with the second bus then you stay with the driver," my mother fretted. "Don't let her leave you on the side of the road in the middle of nowhere."

"She's not going to leave me, Mum, she's got a bus full of special kids. She's not exactly going to leave them on the side of the road."

"You've got your lunch?" she asked me. "Some money just in case? Change for the phone?"

"I'll be all right, Mum," but I was not sure if this was true. I wondered what kind of first impression I would make—fat, nerdy girl from the western suburbs. I imagined the other students all fresh off their farms, fit and healthy and competent at ball sports, already capable of navigating their way through thick bushland, adept at wood chopping and fence building, up and milking the cows before setting out their school uniforms.

All of my references to country kids had come from old musicals, *Paint Your Wagon*, *Seven Brides for Seven Brothers*, *Annie Get Your Gun*. When the bus arrived I kissed my mother quickly.

She talked to the driver, a round, happy woman with curly hair who waved to me and listened closely as my mother recounted her plan for a breakdown "—she can call me from your place, if that's all right. It won't happen, but just in case."

"We'll be fine," the driver winked at me. "Won't we, Krissy?"

"Kris." I wanted to be taken seriously. At Toolooah High in Gladstone I would be arriving with a clean slate. I would remain cautious, speak when spoken to, pretend that I was popular at the last school, leave behind the reek of the nerdy girl. The next three years had the potential to pass with relative ease. Or not.

There were three other kids on the bus, all younger than me. Two of them sat quietly rocking into their reflections on opposite sides of the bus. A Down syndrome boy named Toby grinned from his seat beside the driver. He told me his name and asked for mine. He tried to unclip his seatbelt and shake my hand. The driver grabbed him by the waistband of his shorts and made him sit back down next to her. He grinned and waved and when I waved back he made faces and stuck out his tongue in a way that made me laugh.

There were other kids to collect on the way, a couple of sullen young boys kicking their bags to the back of the bus with all the force their attitude could muster. The bus stopped and a blond girl with a big smile clambered aboard and grinned almost as broadly as Toby.

"Well, hello there," she said and held out her hand for me to shake.

She was pretty in a slouching, wholesome girl-next-door kind of way, and her name was Emily. She was two years younger than me but she drove a truck on the farm and she was just like Annie in *Annie Get Your Gun*. She chatted away to me about her brothers and the farm and the rodeo that was coming up. The rodeo ball was something that I shouldn't miss, apparently; she talked about the boys smelling of bulls and sweat and winked at me as if it was a secret we shared. She had a list of rock stars that she loved, and she was very fond of television. I had nothing in common with her, but she made me laugh and when I told her about Dragonhall, about my family, she said she was dying to meet them and I believed her.

"You should come over for a sleepover," she said.

"I'm not allowed out of the house except for school."

She thought about this and then shrugged. "Well, you'd better invite me over for a sleepover instead. You've got a video player?" We did. "We could have a movie night. I'll bring some vids. We'll make popcorn. I can meet your folks."

She continued on in the special school bus, which would take her right past the Catholic school that she was enrolled at. I waved goodbye as I clambered onto the larger school bus, waiting at the Boyne Island turn-off.

I had made a friend. Already. It seemed impossible, but as I watched her waving to me out of the back window of the minibus I felt that it must be true. My first Queensland friend. A sleepover planned and I hadn't even set foot in the schoolyard.

The school was little, low set, sprawling over hilly lawn. It was very green and there were trees. I tried not to make eye contact with anyone, but they all seemed to want to smile or wave at me. I distrusted their friendliness out of habit and I sat on an empty bench near one wall. A tall, skinny girl with big teeth and the edgy frightened energy of a rabbit sat at the other end of the bench. Another new girl. I knew this because she was wearing a different uniform, a blue check dress from another school.

She grinned shyly in my direction and her whole face was overtaken by the darkest blush. I smiled back, but I refused to speak to her. At my old school she would be the girl that I would sit with, the awkward, intellectual type, prone to being picked on. I cruelly hoped that someone more ordinary would come up to talk to me, someone with the potential to raise me up into a more popular crowd. I was sick of clinging to the rejects and the nerds. Surely I could sneak up the social ladder if I played my cards right. Not the most popular group of course, but just something in the middle ground, a group of kids less likely to get beaten up at lunchtime.

The bell rang and I followed the milling herd into a large auditorium. They seemed to know where they were going and I let them lead me. We all sat cross-legged on the cold concrete floor and the toothy girl sat herself beside me.

"Sheep," she whispered and I noticed her accent, a pinched New Zealand twang on the vowels. "Have you ever wondered what would happen if you got a group of kids to walk the wrong way when the bell rings? Everyone would just follow them. We could make them all walk out into the carpark, sit down next to the cars."

Oh dear. I grinned; of course she was going to be my friend. Cynical, witty, smart as a tack. She was perfect.

"We could herd them over to the Catholic school," I told her. "Get them to sing morning hymns."

"The pool," she whispered, only with her accent it sounded like "pull," and as a teacher climbed up onto the podium and the kids began to settle into silence she added, "Synchronized swimming," which made me splutter into my hand. She was blushing terribly, a beacon, a flare to direct the attention of the unkind kids in our direction, but I resigned myself to it. I would never be with the cool kids but I would enjoy this odd New Zealand girl's company so much more.

Her name was Jenny; we met for recess and lunch and the other kids circled but no one actually threatened us, and I was surprised. There was no confrontation. We survived the first day intact and when we parted company at the front gate I knew that she was just as surprised as I was that we had escaped without the anticipated abuse.

"I might get through the rest of high school without getting my head beaten in," she said. "Imagine surviving till university without thug-inflicted brain damage."

CRUSH

I told Emily about John. I sat next to him; we both played clarinet in the band and there were his beautiful, delicate fingers on the keys. His clarinet case was always neat and perfectly ordered. I threw my reeds in, split and stained with chips knocked out of the finely shaved wood. He cleaned his metal keys until they shone. I hid the crusty verdigris under sweaty fingers. I was a mess.

We sat in class and listened and I could see him following the rise and swell of the music with that intensity that still moves me in a lover. The kind of monofocus that obliterates the real world for the duration. There was also his shy humor, the delicate arrogance of youth. And then there was the weight of my virginity.

I'm not sure when my daydreaming tripped over from the thought of him leaning across my shoulders to help me with my fingering, to the thought of him naked, prizing my virgin panties down over my thighs. This was the pre-sex kind of sexual tension, ripe with possibilities that can never eventuate in any physical beginning. I stopped sleeping. Refused to eat. I lost four dress sizes in six months. Sex rumbled in my belly like a tapeworm and I knew myself, at sixteen, to be capable of obsession. By the time I asked him and he turned me down there was barely anything left of me at all.

In the meantime I told Emily about him and she told me about the roadhouse where she worked and the truckers who stopped there and how sometimes she met them after work and the things they did. She was younger than me. I counted back the years and realized that I would have been assembling the plastic model of the Millennium Falcon when she was climbing into trucks with people's fathers. She talked about muscle and hair and, in the way she told it, these attributes became desirable. She talked about sweat and the smell of diesel and about men, real men, not the kind of clarinet-playing, Dungeons & Dragons boys that I liked.

Every day when Emily climbed onto the bus I would shuffle over and we would lean into each other and there would be my stories of longing and her stories of consummation. She was brave and bold and adventurous. I was all dreaming. When she placed her hand on my knee the heat of her palm burned up and into my groin.

I invited her to my house. I would never be allowed to visit hers.

She had a father and a brother and my family would not let me stay in a house where there would be men. Strange men that could not be trusted. But she was welcome to visit, to sleep over. She brought some videotapes and we dragged a mattress into the lounge room and shuffled across to let the dogs curl around our feet. She had taped *Video Hits* off the television and I watched and listened. At first I didn't like the music, which was poppy and jangly and brash, but when Emily sang along, the songs gained a kind of exuberant energy. We pressed rewind and I learned how to sing the choruses and we stood up on the mattress and danced and she held my hand.

We lounged back against the pillows and I whispered about my longing for John the clarinet player, but with her beside me the longing seemed less directional, more general. She commiserated with me. She touched my hand and I relaxed into the joy of this new kind of sharing.

She slipped another video into the player; a musical. I had my own musicals to watch, I liked *Singing in the Rain*, but I watched *Gentlemen Prefer Blondes* more. I sometimes practiced being Marilyn in front of the mirror, holding her pose, enjoying the generous curves of my body in the way Marilyn might have done, posing, moving, leaning, blowing myself a kiss.

Emily's musical was *The Rocky Horror Picture Show*. It took Marilyn's primping and preening and amplified it. I watched under the covers in the dark and there was the heat of Emily's body so close to mine and sometimes she reached out to me and held me by the shoulders and mouthed the words of a song, a love song, a sex song, and it was all I could do not to touch her in return.

At some point she stopped the tape and made me stand and taught me the dance steps to a particular song and it was all about hips and tits and a slow pelvic grinding. Perhaps I didn't care about the clarinet boy. Perhaps I didn't need to suffer from an unrequited longing.

When the film was over, she slipped in her *Video Hits* tape and turned the volume down so the pop songs became lullabies. We lay side by side and she edged closer to me.

"If I were gay I wouldn't be ashamed of it. I would be out and proud."

"Yes," I told her. "If I liked women I would kiss them in public."

"Hold hands at school."

"I'd tell my family without any angst."

"Maybe I wouldn't tell my brother," she said, "but I'd go live with the girl I loved. And I'd have a wedding. I'd have a *Rocky Horror* wedding and everyone would wear fishnet stockings."

We laughed and we settled more comfortably onto the mattress and I heard her breathing soften into tiredness, and I forced my breath to keep pace with hers. Her hand was between our bodies and I could feel the heat of her fingers almost touching my thigh. I shifted my leg slightly and there was the brush of her fingertips. I imagined that she must be awake, too. I could feel the thud of my heart and the thunder of it should be rocking the mattress. It was certainly shaking my body. My leg would be trembling to the rhythm of it. She would feel it through the tip of her fingers. I reached out the palm of my hand till I could feel the heat off her chest, not close enough to touch her, but close enough to hold her body heat. I clamped my thighs together as my stomach succumbed to that wonderful weightless surge that I associate with desire.

It took most of the night for me to move my finger in slow increments toward her pajama top, and when it was within reach, I touched it. Not hard enough to feel the body beneath, but I could feel the fabric, and the sensation energized me. I was high with it, wakeful. I opened my eyes occasionally, imagining that sooner or later I would find that her eyes were open, too. I played out the scene, a sustained stare, a leaning into each other, a kiss. A fumbling under each other's pajama tops.

"If I were gay I would slip my finger inside you," I would say, slipping my finger inside her.

"If I were gay I would lick your breast." Licking my breast.

The scenario was played out in every possible way and ended each time with us lying in each other's arms, covered in sweat, fingers entwined.

The morning found us at arm's length. Her fingers still barely grazing my thigh, my fingers almost touching her breast. I was stiff and sore and exhausted from such a wakeful night. She opened her eyes and stretched and turned and I felt a surge of regret. When she stood and asked if there was coffee I felt the cold morning air slide in under the blankets.

"Yes. Coffee would be good," I said.

LEAVING

My sister was a stranger by then.

She had worked for a while in the corner store but she returned home and shut her door and stayed there with the curtains drawn and Pink Floyd turned up loud. Sometimes when I passed her in the corridor she glared at me with such hatred that I began to wonder if she would be likely to kill me in my sleep. I imagined waking up with a pillow over my face and no chance to shout for help.

On better days she would venture out and sit in front of a video and perhaps even speak to me. I was careful with my conversations because she was prone to sudden rages. She would shriek and throw things and then, as if a switch had been thrown, she would suddenly power down. All signs of life gone. She would sit in complete silence, her eyes shut or open, and I would tiptoe around her, worried, but cautious as well, in case I somehow reactivated her.

Her friend from school made the long trip up north to visit and for a while I could see my sister again. The smart playful girl who was fond of setting challenges and forcing you to participate.

When he left I saw the life draining out of her. She took her paints into her bedroom and concentrated on making intricate dark pictures of buff knights and vampire women. Sex oozing out of the images. She would have to leave. I knew she would have to leave.

She applied for university without telling anyone.

I emerged from a restless Christmas break, thin from a regime of starvation, tanned from days of walking back and forth along the access road, and when I glanced into my sister's room I noticed the difference immediately. She was packed and ready to leave us.

The idea of leaving home was complicated. My aunt never had left home. My mother, in the brief time that she had tried to venture away from the nest, had barely settled. She'd spent most evenings at my grandmother's, walking between houses with her children in tow. My grandmother exerted an incredible pull, like some vast astrological body, dragging everything in the universe toward her. My mother was sucked back into her orbit but once there she was kept at arm's length, punished for her small foray out into the world, never again to be accepted back into the idea of home.

Karen would go, and then she would be gone. My mother spent

her evenings in tears. She knew the price you had to pay for leaving home. Maybe Karen could do her degree through distance education; she could send her assignments by mail. These were the options that could save her from the ultimate sin of leaving.

My sister used the glamour of a university degree to slip away. My mother had graduated from teachers' college. My aunt went to tech. Karen would be the first person in the family to be awarded a Bachelor of Arts.

I went back to school. I sat on the bus with Emily and spent my days mooning over the boy with the clarinet. I was voted school captain and I knew that I was a compromise. The teachers liked me because I was pleasant, honest, and compliant. The students chose me because I didn't really care. They could smoke in the toilets and I wouldn't report them. No one really hated me, but they didn't like me either. I auditioned for the school musical and won the starring role. And then, one day, my sister left.

I could have her room if I wanted it. It was larger than mine and painted a dark and moody purple. There were black sheets. She had left her collection of fantasy novels and I could read them, but I didn't really want to. I wrote to her once but she didn't reply. She called home dutifully but there was a distance in the conversations. Her answers were monosyllabic. I wondered how it would be to leave. I knew I would never be brave enough, but maybe I would.

I stood on the stage and sang about love and kissed the leading boy and it was my first kiss. Out there in public, in front of an audience of several hundred, I reached up for his neck and he bent down to my height. He was six foot six, I was five foot one. It was a kind of visual comedy but for me it was real and powerful and I opened my mouth there on the stage. There was an exchange of tongues and when I pulled away I said my line, which was "I love you," and he said "I love you, too." We were performing, but we would repeat the kiss in private at the after-party. I would know that even then, without the audience, we were performing an act, but it was an act that I was excited by. I kissed my leading man and I went home singing with the force of the kiss and told my mother that I had been asked on a date—even though, in reality, I had asked him.

ABANDONING THE HYMEN

The brush I had been using was tiny, a few sable hairs bound together. Like underwear, paintbrushes are more expensive the smaller they are. I was making fiddly adjustments to a lead figurine of a man in a tunic with high boots and a sword at his hip, adjusting the color of his cape while we waited on my aunt so the game could begin. My mother spent the time re-reading the adventure we were about to go on. "Into the Spider Lands," or something equally appealing—these Dungeon modules were all the same. It was like reading a crime novel or a romance, a pattern that rarely wavered from its course. By now I felt I had outgrown these family adventures anyway, but tomorrow I would be losing my virginity and there was something comforting in the idea of gaming with my family.

I blew on the little metal figure until the paint dried and told my mother how my first date was going to be conducted. She was going to drive me the hour it would take to get to Gladstone, then she would wait for me at a safe distance. I told her I was old enough.

"Next year I will be gone," I said, knowing suddenly that it was true and that it would be fine. "Next year I will go to university like my sister."

She cried, and I hated to see her cry, but I refused to budge. I refused to scramble back into the safe nest that my grandmother had made for us. I would go on my date and I would leave home and, out on my own, everything would be okay.

Tim made me buy the condoms.

"You're the one who wants to have sex," he told me. "You buy the condoms." Which seemed only fair until I was standing at the counter with a packet of Durex in my hand. I thought the chemist could smell my hymen. I had that whiff of virginity about me. I wanted it to be the woman who served me, but of course it was the man, and I met his eyes as I handed him the packet. I stared directly into his eyes as if my heart wasn't thudding out my panic. I didn't even know what condoms looked like really. I didn't really know what a penis would look like either.

I had already felt his penis through his trousers. I had felt it in the cinema, my hand sneaking over the armrest, spilling popcorn into my own lap, shivery fingers into his. I touched it and learned that it was apparently of impossible dimensions. Even my longest fattest candle at home didn't seem quite so long and thick. I had never anticipated putting something so big inside my body, but the hymen must be broken somehow. I made Tim pay half the money because surely that was fair and I stood at the counter and eyeballed the middle-aged man and silently dared him to ask me anything about my purchase of those condoms.

"I bought the condoms," I told him, looking up. He played basketball and hung around a group of boys who also played basketball. His best friend was even taller than he was, and sweeter, nicer to be around. This did not bother me. I had kissed my leading man and therefore I would sleep with him.

Before our first kiss, the stage kiss, we had barely said a word to each other outside rehearsals. Tim liked to play sports. I liked to play the clarinet and Dungeons & Dragons. There was no possible subject for a conversation between us, and yet here we were, kissing, and the heat of that kiss traveled down into my stomach and settled there, butting against my hymen like a demon child desperate to be released from its cage.

The plan was that we would have sex on the beach while my mother waited for me in the car, since I couldn't travel anywhere without her. She would wait just within shouting distance, making sure that I could not get into any trouble. My mother knew that this was a date and that

I was here with a boy. I had my one-piece bathing suit on under my jeans and T-shirt. He was wearing boardshorts. We would swim. I argued that I needed some small moment of privacy, just time alone to talk and perhaps hold hands. I'm not sure if I promised her that nothing would happen but I might have.

I was determined to abandon my hymen on that beach in the light of day. I had a patterned towel because I knew there might be some blood. I had read about this, small drops of red on a wedding sheet, hung out for all the villagers to cheer over; rose petals of color on the virgin white panties of some fallen girl. I had the condoms in my pocket and I had purchased them without any assistance. Nothing, not even my own promises or the presence of my mother, was going to stop me from executing my task.

I took his hand and plummeted. I ran down the beach and around the curve of ocean to where my mother wouldn't see me disappearing into the scrubby strand with Tim the basketball player trailing from my hand like a huge kite. He caught the wind and dragged at me, but I tugged against him. There was very little time. In a matter of minutes my mother would be strolling along the sand, peering out into the ocean, looking for the little bobbing buoys of our heads.

His penis was very large. That was my first and only thought. I watched it spring up from his boardshorts like a little white flag, marking a place in the center of his wiry pubic hair. I thought about golf. I knew he played golf.

I checked my watch and undressed hurriedly, wrangled condoms. They seemed too small. I wrestled one out of its packet and it was a skinny limp skin. Shriveled, miserable.

"Do they come in sizes?" he asked me.

"I don't know. How do I know?"

"Didn't you ask?"

I thought of the old man behind the counter at the chemist, handed Tim the droop of latex, watched him scrabble with his ridiculous protrusion. Time was ticking on. My mother would be sitting on a bench pretending to read her book, watching the ocean and waiting for me to drift into view. He tried and failed to do anything useful with the condom; it dropped into the prickly grass at his feet.

Only five condoms left now. The thought that I might return home still a virgin was intolerable.

"Here, I'll do it," I said.

I pulled another little rubber worm from the packet, and the hot sand scratched against my knees.

Who was to know there would be so much blood?

And it hurt. He looked down at me for a moment; he paused and asked if he should stop, but we pushed on. The condom seemed too tight and I had not yet learned about lubrication. I was dry and there was sand and we were running to a deadline. I had to check my watch from time to time and listen for the squeak of my mother's feet on the sand.

When the hymen broke it was a painful relief. The blood began to flow, which eased the chafing, but I didn't even attempt an orgasm. The job was done: I was ready to down tools and head off to the pub for a beer. But the blood was everywhere and I wondered how I would be able to hide it. My white swimsuit would be ruined, the towel was a mess of sand and gore. Then Tim rolled the condom off and there was only half of it left. The rest had disappeared mysteriously somewhere inside me. Blood and semen then. I wanted to cry.

"What if you get pregnant?" he groaned. "What if I've got the school captain pregnant?"

I had a name. He knew it but he chose to see me as I had never seen myself, as a rank, the captain of the school that he attended. I looked at him then, this sports-playing giant of a boy. I was grateful for the removal of my hymen but suddenly, for the first time, I wondered if I should have waited for someone I cared about.

"I won't get pregnant."

"How do you know?"

"I'll get the morning after pill."

This seemed to satisfy him. He leaned over and kissed me. I accepted the kiss without pleasure. I was planning things, crossing them off an imaginary list. Get dressed, hide the towel drenched in blood, tell my mother I needed to go to the doctor. Tell her that I was old enough, that she didn't have to come with me. Why did she always come in to the doctor with me? I had just turned eighteen and therefore I was a woman and I could see the doctor by myself. There would be a fight, it would end in tears. I would have to tell her outright. That's what I should do.

"Mother, I've just had sex and I need the morning after pill," I would say. Just like that. Quick, and all the pain would be over, just like the breaking of the hymen.

The boy was talking to me. I looked at him, tried to focus. I should listen to this tall and sporty boy who had just lost his own virginity to me. I should take an interest. I gazed at him, this boy I barely knew and didn't particularly like, and nothing he said could be of interest to me. I closed my eyes and lay back in the sand, gathering my strength for our departure.

GONE

I knew I would miss the place terribly. I didn't want to leave. I had made friends. There was Emily and the evenings we still spent bemoaning the fact that we weren't gay, lying next to each other, and me with my secret desire spilling over onto her side of the bed, my fingers touching her hip as she slept, my nostrils flaring toward that particularly delightful sleeping-girl smell.

I would miss sharing meals with my grandmother and my aunt, the early mornings lazing at the breakfast table drinking the perfect pot of leaf tea. Eating freshly cooked bread hot from the oven.

I would miss those infrequent moments with my grandfather at the piano, while my grandmother huffed and puffed and moaned about the noise hurting her head. I would miss the menagerie, all the animals that I helped to groom and care for.

I would miss James, the new boy who had started to drive the long distance out to our property to spend afternoons with me playing video games and play-fighting and stealing stray moments to touch. He would leave with the scent of me on his fingers and on his lips. I would spend my evenings restlessly longing for his next visit, or for Emily, to talk to about his next visit.

There was all of November, December, and January after the end of the school year and I spent my days writing a novel which I finished just before I had to leave for university. It was a story of unrequited love, of traveling, moving on, and leaving people behind. It was set on a strange planet where magic happens. There were echoes of Dragonhall in its pages although I could not see it then.

I did not let them see me cry. I didn't want to leave. I wanted to cancel my enrollment or defer. I wanted to stay home, unchanging, to remain a part of the family. My grandmother hugged me stiffly. She rarely hugged and it seemed uncomfortable for her to do so. She was dry eyed and tight-lipped and I knew I was a disappointment.

"Be good girl. Don't do what I would do."

"Don't do what she wouldn't do," Sheila corrected. My aunt and my grandmother. I would never again be as close to them as I was at that moment, and I knew this as I hugged them. When I turned to my mother she was crying.

"I love you," I told her. "I'll miss you."

And it was true.

A PLAN

Brisbane 2008

By the time I am forty I will have my first novel published. By the time I am forty I will have lost weight. By the time I am forty I will have developed a calm wisdom and will spend a large part of every day helping younger people to find that wisdom, too. I will have abandoned my sudden inexplicable flashes of jealousy, and I will have become beautiful. I will achieve these goals.

If I have not achieved these goals then I will climb to the top of the Story Bridge. I will drink a bottle of champagne by myself, knowing that it was not from want of trying. I will step over the rails and hang there, enjoying the beauty of the lights of the city reflected in the river. At the end of the drop there will be the relief of knowing that I will not have to struggle so hard anymore. I will not be scrambling like a rat in a wheel, desperate to keep myself up and away from the terrible bottoming out that will be back and back and back again.

At the bottom of things I am unkind to myself. I will fall onto the water as if it were concrete, and when the weight of me drags this body under the surface the undertow will be gentle and I will be carried quietly away from myself.

"It's like I am setting myself up," I tell the counselor as she sits and closes her eyes. I wonder if she might be bored and nodding into a deep sleep. "I choose someone who will not be attracted to me and I develop this obsession so that they can tell me I am unattractive and cannot be loved."

She opens her eyes. She is tired but she is awake.

"Ah," she says. "So maybe this is not about sex at all."

I am not following her. I am tired and harried and confused. "But it is about sex," I tell her. "I always want to have sex with them. I dream I am having sex."

She looks at her watch.

"Same time next week?"

Another week and then another and then I will be forty.

I hear about someone I know just a little who has taken his own life on his fortieth birthday. Quietly slipped away to a place where he will no longer be in pain. I am overcome by a wave of jealous anger. How can I follow through with my plan now? Now I will seem derivative. I read about the suicide of David Foster Wallace and everyone is sad, it seems, except me.

"Maybe he was just fed up," I tell Christopher.

I watch him bend to retrieve the cash from the safe and find that I am no longer overwhelmed by that sudden rush of lust. I am both relieved and disappointed. The sink is still overflowing and I haven't found another bucket to catch the water. I feel it spill onto the floor and am overwhelmingly sad. I realize that although I have cruised through my little infatuations, it has been a long time since anyone showed any interest in me. I stare tiredly into the mirror and quite frankly, I can see their point.

I was sitting in a pub the other day and a man came up to me. He was a short man, inoffensive. He was wearing a yellow reflective jacket like a tradie or a cyclist. He was old—my age, I reminded myself, which is old. I looked up from my book, bleary eyed, emerging from a good story well told.

"Can I sit here?"

There were seats everywhere. The bar was almost empty but there were a few other girls, prettier girls, girls younger than me and he had picked me out because I looked old and single and perhaps lonely.

"I mean, is this seat taken? Do you mind if I sit here?"

He looked fine. Not mentally ill or drunk or high on anything as far as I could tell. He wanted to sit with me and chat, just a quiet conversation after work. No one has tried to pick me up in years. I am tempted to say that no one has ever tried to pick me up, but that would be wrong. There was one boy who asked me on a date and there were those two drunken men who chased me at 2:00 AM one night.

I suppose that was a come-on of sorts. But really, in the scheme of things, there has been no one interested.

This one was interested. Tentative. Interested. I looked at him, mole blind from the book, a little sad from the one glass of wine drunk too quickly.

If I were single now, there would be no men plucked from my furtive fantasies, no wild affairs with those young men I fall in lust with slowly, one at a time. If I were single those same young men would not sit and have a beer with me after work. I could perhaps go back to my life of casual sex and one-night stands. There would be some pleasure in it I suppose.

The first and only pick-up. This possibly nice man who is possibly the same age as me or maybe a little older.

I refuse politely. I have my book to finish, my good story well told. I have a second glass of wine to consume it with. I have my fruitless infatuations with people half the age that I am now. I have my secret masturbatory fantasies. I have a husband, shielding me from the harsh glare of reality, from the horrible potential of quietly following this man, who is as old and sad as I am, back to his lonely bed.

He doesn't insist. He excuses himself politely and I watch out of the corner of my eye as he stands at the bar and quietly finishes his beer and walks out and away, rejected. Dejected.

And my heart breaks just a little, for his sake, but mostly for my own.

THE SAFETY
OF CUPBOARDS

Brisbane 1987

I stood under a streetlight in the middle of the throng, clutching my map. I was in Brisbane, the Queen Street Mall, and there were people everywhere. There were groups of them, giggling couples holding hands, rangy tribes of teenagers hooting to each other across a sea of heads. My coat still held a hint of popcorn and Maltesers in its folds, the scent of the cinema. Strange to be standing in the dark, when I had entered the cinema in the glare of daylight: my first day in the city. I was alone and out in the world.

Alone. I had never been alone like this. I stood at the bus stop and realized I had never bought a ticket for myself. I had never read a timetable. I had never sat in the movies without someone beside me. I turned the map over in my hands, matching my direction against the street signs. I had never had to follow a map before. I had been ferried from home to school to the shops and home again. I had never been responsible for my own direction. Now I was free. Free to go anywhere. I was free.

In fact, I was going to the Country Women's Association hostel my mother had arranged for me. Eventually I found the street and walked it.

The building was old and tall, impressive in the way that hospitals or homes for the mentally ill are impressive. There was a dining area on the ground floor. Girls were sitting in groups, girls eating or watching television. Girls laughing and whispering and glancing up at me, the stranger in their midst. They could smell my difference. They heard it in my accent and saw it written on my sallow skin. They nodded to me in the elevator but I noticed how the conversation suddenly fell away. I heard the sound of it start up when I slunk down the corridor to my room. My room was gray and small, a desk sunk into one corner, a bed skulking in another. The wall-to-ceiling cupboard was finished in a wood veneer, the warmest thing in the place.

I lay on the bed and the springs creaked. There was a sign in the lobby warning that men, including members of the family, were not allowed past the dining room. The creaking springs seemed like a secondary alarm. No tossing or turning or petting of any kind. I imagined they wouldn't expect the girls to put the springs to the test with each other. The CWA did not anticipate the idea of love between girls, or else they shrugged it off.

I lay on the bed and listened to the steady creak in time to my breathing. I switched the bedside light on. Gray shadows slicing geometric shapes out of a gray room, monochrome. Gray on gray on gray. A deafening palette blended out of white and black. I pulled the novel out from under my pillow and tried to read. Black writing on white paper. Black and white and all of it gray.

I pulled the duvet off the bed and opened the door of the cupboard. A small cramped space, but large enough for me to make a nest. It was dark in the cupboard, and safe, and the wood was fast against the wall, no creaking springs. I wriggled out of my pajamas. I touched myself for comfort and it was comforting, but briefly. When I was finished there was still the gray room outside and the sounds of the city and the first night alone. First night ever alone.

I dragged the oversized speaker box toward the cupboard. It was an easy thing to climb up onto the box. I had to drag myself up on tiptoe, balancing against the cupboard door. I hooked my arms through the upper reaches of the door frame and heaved myself up, scrabbling awkwardly on the lip of the top shelf.

When I was finally up there it was cozier than the bottom of the cupboard. There were pillows and extra blankets. I was safe, and suddenly terribly tired. I cried from tiredness, soft tears with no force behind them. I missed my family. I missed my home, my jail. I was finally free and I wished I was not. I longed for chains and rules and the smother of love. I pressed my face against the pillow. There was no air, and there I was hoping that I might drown in this tiny space above the cupboard. And slowly, breath by shallow breath, I fell asleep.

I woke into a predawn moment, entombed. It was cold and cramped and one of my legs was numb.

I could hear the traffic, the oceanic swell, and I knew that I was not at home. First night away from home. I was homesick for the press of dogs around my knees, warm damp fur bodies, the smell of caged birds, the crushing love of my family.

I had survived the night and took a fierce pride in it. I shifted awkwardly and shook my foot; felt the painful prickle of blood rushing back. Despite the general family consensus that I would have difficulty surviving in the world, I was still here. I had seen a movie by myself. I had walked home. I had rested, after a fashion.

I shrugged the night off, swinging my legs out so that I was hanging off the high ledge of the cupboard like a terracotta angel, and I realized then how far it would be to the floor.

The speaker box was there beneath me. It was just a matter of turning in this cramped place, bracing myself in the structure of the cupboard with my arms, elbows splayed, then lowering myself onto the tall rectangle of wood. From there, it was a simple thing to slip onto the floor.

I sat on the precarious ledge for what seemed like a long time. The sound of traffic filled out. Tide coming in, commuters rising, showering, dressing. There was a peal of laughter from somewhere down the corridor. Girls gathered, running toward the lift and down to breakfast in the communal dining place where boys were allowed but not encouraged, and I was stranded.

I would find pictures, I thought. I would hang them above my desk and day by day they would spread across the walls, creeping over toward the bed and into my dreams. I would pick flowers. I would have no money to buy flowers, but I would pluck them from fence lines and pop them into a water bottle on the desk. I would search for flowers with a scent, jasmine, mock orange, to bring some pleasure to a lifeless space. I would fill the room with music to dispel the ache of emptiness. And, more important, I would find bodies to touch mine. I would be naked with someone new. I would provide my flesh with a distraction.

But first I had to climb down out of the cupboard.

In my particular family folklore, the one that families invent for you, I am clumsy and I am vague. I have barely a toe on the earth and the rest of me is lost to the atmosphere. "That's Krissy," they would say when I spilled a tepid puddle from a cup of tea or forgot my sentence halfway though. And it was with this fabled clumsiness that I executed a halting turn, edging my bottom toward the perilous drop. There was nowhere to lodge my fingers. I hooked my elbows around the door frame. There was nothing to do that would lessen the risk of plummeting. I took slow sure breaths. I would have one chance at this dismount. I tightened the muscles in my arms and this was my support. I crawled to the very edge and then there was the clean jerk of my body falling, but I was safe, held up by my arms. I searched about for the edge of the speaker box and my probing foot set it to listing back and forth, a precarious balance. I could feel the shudder in my arms and the slow burn of effort. I was light. I was as slight as I had ever been, thinned down by a stubborn refusal to eat. I was light, but there was no muscle to hold me there. I rested a toe on the speaker box. I would have to let go and there would be a small fall in this, but I would be perched in safety. I could visualize the result. I held my breath and let go.

The speaker box slipped and I fell. Felt a flash of pain. Then nothing.

I woke to the sound of cars, fewer of them now, the rush hour long gone. How long? There was still pain. I felt it in my scalp, waves of it, washing over me. I was in an ocean of the stuff and it was difficult to breathe, but I did, small shuddering breaths. So I had fallen. Had I broken something? My leg or my back? Perhaps I had snapped my spine. I certainly felt as if it would be impossible to move. With difficulty I reached down my body. I was wet, it felt as if I had wet myself. I touched the damp fabric at my crotch and the pain exploded, new and all consuming. My hand came away damp, but not with urine.

There was blood; I peeled down my pajama pants and there

was so much blood there on my thighs. Somehow when I slipped I had caught the edge of the speaker box in my crotch. My vulva was horribly torn, my clitoris swollen to the size of a small orange.

My first panicked thought was of sex. I had destroyed the possibility of pleasure. I thought about life without the relief of an orgasm and knew I would rather be dead. I wondered if I could somehow develop the ability to have nonclitoral orgasms, the fabled vaginal ones that I had read about. I wondered about reconstructions, plastic surgery, a stitching-up of ruined flesh and the softer skin taken from the back of my neck or my elbow.

I lay awake in the pain for what seemed like a mess of days. Somehow, eventually, I would have to move; and so I did. I dragged myself along the carpet as though it were an assault course. I kamikaze-crawled. I butted up against the door and there it was like a mountain, something to be conquered. Somehow I managed to drag myself to my knees without fainting. I stretched for the door handle and miraculously it was in my hand, and the door was open. I was sprawled in the corridor and there was no one about and there was the lift at the other end and I had to crawl to it. I imagined ants dragging twigs hundreds of times larger than themselves. I thought of maggots, hatched and wriggling, seemingly on the spot, babies burning their skin on carpet, grunting their frustration, edging toward tears.

The elevator doors opened and the girl inside screamed. It must have looked as if I had been stabbed. She saw the blood and she shrieked.

Then she pulled me into the elevator and I relaxed into her panicked care. We were somehow in the lobby. I was kneeled beside, I was tended to. I sank into the hurt and the embarrassment of it all. They asked me what happened and I was not sure how to say that I was sleeping in the top of a cupboard without sounding like a freak. I was a freak. The ambulance drivers glanced at each other and I knew that it must be bad. I was thinking—I will never have sex ever again. I will never have an orgasm. I will die now. Must die. They gave me painkillers and I became drowsy and it still hurt, but I was distanced from it.

In the hospital the doctors came in packs and looked but didn't touch. The swelling had grown to the size of a baseball, a purple black canker.

The same question: "How did this happen?"

I invented a complex story about spring-cleaning, the same fall described in detail but with a different prologue. I knew that they could feel the lie. I was unused to lying. This invention, this half truth, was a new thing for me. They knew there was something amiss and so they held me, feeding me painkillers, trooping through the ward and asking me to keep my legs spread (as if I could have clamped them together in my present state). It occurred to me that they believed I had been abused. One nurse asked me about my living situation, my boyfriend. I had no boyfriend, or no one currently in the same city as myself. I thought about James, the boy from Gladstone, who wrote to me and told me he would wait for me. He would always love me.

"I fell out of a cupboard," I told them again and again, and it must have sounded like "I ran into the door," or "I slipped down the stairs." It was a lie in its unlikeliness.

When a week was up they released me into the world. I had enough money for a cab fare but I would have no money for phone calls home or bus fares or food when I got there.

I hobbled to the hostel on crutches. I slept in the bottom of the cupboard with the speaker box murmuring a classical lullaby. Bach. I had a sudden longing for my grandfather and his piano and I took the tape out of the machine and replaced it with a mix tape, songs of sadness and longing. Love is a stranger of a different kind, ground control to Major Tom, Heathcliffe, it's me, I'm Cathy, I've come home.

The bruising faded, the swelling eased back to a kind of normalcy. After a time I began to masturbate, carefully, in my cupboard nest. No response at first, but slowly my body responded to my touch. A gentle climax. A slow return to form. The orgasms eased the loneliness a little. I abandoned the crutches. I found myself restless in the evenings and I left the confines of my student prison to wander the streets of Spring Hill.

The houses were beautiful. The beautiful people in them had city lives full of excitement and families and friends. Everyone was busy doing something of importance, it seemed. I glimpsed them through half-drawn curtains. I passed them spilling out from the doorways of pubs. I came to know the streetwalkers by sight. I ventured to the edges of parks. I stood under the glow of streetlights and was bathed in otherworldliness. There were mad people pacing and talking to themselves and wandering in endless circles down streets, up streets, around streets. I passed the same man several times and suddenly realized that from his perspective it might have been me who was mad and aimless. I sat in my lonely gray room with the flowers sagging under the weight of days, petals dropping in time to the rhythmless strains of early Pink Floyd. I became restless quickly and I was back to walking. Time passed and passed and passed some more.

DRAG AND THE DRAMA QUEEN

Brisbane 2008

My brother-in-law pulls a photograph out of his wallet. It is a picture of a girl in a bikini. She is pretty in a glossy-magazine kind of way. Long legs, blond hair cascading down a perfectly tanned back. No cellulite anywhere on her body, no stretchmarks, a breezy summer face. He shows the photograph to the boys, his brothers. My husband leans over and takes the photo out of his hand. They are alike in some ways, the three brothers. They are tall and share strong features, chiseled jaws, long bones. En masse they are impressive, like young stags, sparring, locking horns, showing off. The three of them nod at his photograph, and his other brother rummages in his own wallet. Another photograph, another swimsuit model, this one his own. I glance at the pictures, their beautiful leggy girlfriends, and I feel sad for my husband. No photograph in his wallet, his chubby dark-haired wife slouching back toward the couch where her book is waiting.

There is a photograph of the extended family. The parents, the aunts, the three boys with their respective partners. A summery beachside photograph and all of them grinning in their pastel shirts and shoestring straps and boardshorts. I am the odd one out. I am overdressed, in a black gown. I look like I have been transported there from another planet. I am an alien amongst them, the foreigner. We laugh about this photograph. "One of these things is not like the others," my husband says. I laugh, but I am sad for him, my husband with his attractive family and their attractive extended family, their bikini girlfriends reading their glossy magazines and sunning themselves on deck chairs, and me.

I am approaching my fortieth birthday. I do so with a sad drag of my feet, walking toward the disappointment of my unmet goals. And then there is the dislocation between my appearance and my actions. I feel like a drag queen, strutting a rampant sexuality that is just an overblown façade. Smoke and mirrors and not particularly thick smoke at that.

In the cruel light of day I really can't bear to look at myself. That is the problem with stopping to think about it all. In the moment of sex there is nothing but forward motion. There is pleasure, the active taking of pleasure and then giving back and everything is in motion.

Now, with the light and the stale sheets still damp, there is a pause and I am left with myself and I am ashamed. This is what other women feel, I am sure of it. I see the signs of it in their eyes as they fail to meet my fierce gaze.

In my own head there are indigestible clues.

I walk past a group of boys who sit spotted and ugly in the drunken gutter. I hear one of them howl like a wolf and yell out, "Dog." It is only a moment later that I realize he is referring to me. The moment lodges in my brain like a blood clot.

The fetid drunken homeless man shambles past and looks up at me, blurry eyed, his breath a nightmare as he spits out the word "Fat" and moves on. Another clot forms, throbbing in my temple.

The group of men at the pub who point at me and call out, "There's your girlfriend," and splutter laughter to each other. A hook in my head that could catch fish.

I am unlovely. I am overweight. I am strident and combative. I do not wear matching underwear. I do not wear perfume or makeup or work out in a gym. I have grown older as we all grow older and there are still kids to grow up into that teenage moment of desirability.

I stand amongst the stained sheets wishing it were darker, wishing there was no mirror in the room, wishing there was still flesh pressed up against mine because when it is all kissing and sucking and touching there is no room for looking or pondering over those brain-hemorrhaging kernels of derision lodged in my memory.

UNIVERSITY

Brisbane 1987

I chose to study drama because I didn't want to be a journalist and I couldn't think of another course that would teach me to be a novelist. I could have studied literature, I should have. I chose drama because of the musicals and the first kiss and the idea that there might be more stage kisses that might lead to other things. I chose drama because of the idea of sex.

The drama students reminded me of the peacocks we kept at home. Flamboyant. They regaled each other with loud and theatrical stories during breaks. They leaped up on tables. They all seemed to love Shakespeare and quoted scenes from Shakespearean dramas at every opportunity. I watched, entertained but slightly disquieted. They were all so beautiful. The girls were thin and had clear skin and intelligent eyes. The boys were toned and fit with interesting haircuts. I snapped back into my shell. I was a silent witness to their performances. I was an average student. I couldn't sing my chakras in Voice and Movement like the other students could. I felt silly standing in a circle and feeling the energy of the rest of the group. We all had to leap in the air and say "Ha!" when the energy was right, but I was always a fraction late, responding to the sudden movement of the students rather than some kind of universal force. They spoke about spirituality as if it was a science. They talked about "the muse." I went back to my lonely flat in the evenings and wrote my stories and my poems as I always had and I suspected that there was no muse, there was just a lot of hard work and persistence. I couldn't say this to them.

One day we were sitting in the refectory and they were talking about sex. I had begun to collect the classic texts, Anaïs Nin, Georges Batailles. I read all the books that would have been banned at home. I had a growing appetite for voyeurism. Sometimes in my night wandering I would look through curtainless windows and see people copulating, and I would stand and watch until it was done. I was learning about sex. There was nobody to practice with, but there was a whole world of information churning in my imagination. If the other drama students could talk about sex then so could I. I suspected I could hold my own.

They giggled as they spoke about head jobs, cunnilingus. The forbidden things that their parents had warned them of but they had discovered were more enjoyable than expected. I felt as if, finally, I had adult contact, adult conversation. Nothing could be prohibited in such risqué and exciting company.

"I never expected I would actually enjoy giving a head job," one of them said, blushing slightly but continuing with her bold talk. We were drama students, and sex talk was like that: dramatic and bold.

"Condoms," said one of them and was treated to a deluge of condom stories.

"Orgasms," said another and the orgasm stories rained down.

"Anal sex."

"Oh," I said, "I haven't tried it with a boy, but I like it. Or I like doing it to myself." I laughed. At last I could join in with their bawdy talk. "I like the feel of it. It's more exciting, maybe because of the pain. Maybe that focuses the pleasure." The others just stared at me, in silence. I had overstepped some kind of invisible boundary that I didn't know existed. I needed to back out quickly. "But I haven't tried it with a real person. Only masturbating. Only just a little bit. Not a whole penis, small things, hardly anal sex at all really."

Someone changed the topic. I wanted someone to respond so that I could valiantly defend my stance on anal sex, but they moved on to other things. Put some distance between them and me. I was embarrassed back into silence.

One of the other girls mentioned her new job modeling. Katherine was a sweet girl, luminously beautiful, statuesque with long black curls and porcelain skin. Her family knew artists, not artists like my own mad hermit family, but rich artists who threw proper parties and exhibited in private galleries. Katherine modeled for a few of them and found there was a circuit of modeling to be done.

Back in my cold unloved flat I pored through my collected Anaïs Nin. Stories about artists and their models and the sex between the two, and yes, stories about anal sex and the pleasure that can be had, a pleasure that reflected my own. I suspected that no matter how sophisticated and worldly they seemed, the drama students were wrong, that it was all right to enjoy this kind of physical sensation. That no sensation should be taboo. I thought about my evenings with Emily and *The Rocky Horror Picture Show* and I curled up inside my cupboard, and I masturbated. I inserted a finger into my anus while I did it and enjoyed it despite them.

The problem with taking my clothes off in public was my relationship to my body. It was a young body, not quite nineteen yet. It was tighter than it would be in subsequent years. It was fitter. Drama classes provided a regime of movement that stretched and toned and whittled away the puppy fat. I had started to eat since leaving home, but my diet consisted of small cups of couscous with avocado sliced into it, some tamari, tahini on rice crackers. I ate occasionally and on the run. I couldn't bear to sit amongst the other girls in the Country Women's Association accommodation dining hall. I tended to help myself to an apple and some crackers and cheese, hover at the edge of the dining room, swallow it down with a coffee, before grabbing a coat and racing out into the night. I couldn't bear to be alone in my flat. I walked for miles and sometimes I would stop and fish a novel out of my satchel and curl up under a streetlight to read for a while before wandering off again. My restlessness burned calories.

My body would not look nicer than it did in those days, and yet, when I stepped out of my clothes in front of the students, all I could think about was the dimpling on my thighs, and the midget proportions of my calf bones compared to the rest of me and the soft place on my belly. I undressed in the crowded room because there didn't seem to be anywhere else to do it. I stood naked and faced the students who would be studying my body.

They were art students and this meant there was a lot of cheesecloth in the room. Hairstyles were colorful and full of texture. These students were not as beautiful as my own class, they were thin and pale and beaky, but still they seemed more beautiful than me.

I stared them down. When the lecturer suggested I should do a series of quick twenty-second poses as a warm-up, I made sure to have eye contact with at least one student for each pose. This is how I survived it, that first time. Later it would be easier, but that first time was a challenge and I faced it as such. The room was cold, the students were my own age.

That first time my poses passed without comment. I did what was asked of me and then I dressed hurriedly, took my cash and left the room. I didn't even glance at their sketchbooks. I didn't want to see myself interpreted through their eyes. Later, at another session, a young student whined that they always got fat models and I was mortified and almost quit the job. But he was a pimply, consumptive type with a fringe that covered his eyes and when I looked at his sketch pad he had turned me into a stick figure anyway. His figures were not at all beautiful. I could see his criticism for what it was, he was blaming his tools as any bad artist does. My mother had taught me that on our afternoons painting in front of the television. A bad artist blames the tools. I dressed and walked toward the bad artist at the end of the class, brushing past his mediocre images, making his easel wobble.

Sometimes I posed for Katherine's clients in their big houses with their expensive canvases. I didn't particularly like the work I saw on their walls, but they were rich and I supposed their work must be more valuable than I could judge.

"Pretend you are washing your hair," one of them told me. I raised my hands to my scalp. This is how I washed my hair. It wasn't a particularly interesting pose.

"No, no. Like this." He showed me. Some kind of lean and bend, an athletic kind of personal grooming that I had never seen before. So this is how other people wash their hair, I thought. I am doing it wrong.

I was constantly astonished by the real world. Everything was new and strange. I had never experienced other people's lives. I had never stayed at someone else's house before leaving home, I had never spent quality time with anyone outside of Dragonhall. I entered university trusting blindly that everyone else's way of doing things was probably the way things should be done.

I kept up the modeling, wondering when one of the artists would find me attractive and proposition me, as in Anaïs Nin stories. I waited, and slowly, session after session, began to realize that none of them found me attractive at all.

I wrote to the boy from Gladstone and he wrote back to me. I love you, he told me. I love you, I said back, but I knew I was just speaking from the kind of loneliness that bites into your bones, the kind you could die from unless you found your way out eventually. When I let myself back into the Country Women's Association late at night and rode the elevator to my floor, I felt numb. When I sat on the single bed there and pulled off my sandals I would find that I was crying, and wonder when the tears had started. I would pick them off my cheeks and let them drip from my fingers, curious. I was crying and I knew that probably meant I felt sad, but really I felt nothing at all.

RAYMONT LODGE

John, the boy who played the clarinet, lived across town in a lodge in Auchenflower run by the Uniting Church. I sat quietly with him at a café and I no longer felt all that teenage angst and longing that had plagued me through the years of high school, but it was good to see him again.

He lived in Raymont Lodge, more expensive than my own accommodation and not as close to the university, but I didn't care. I had to leave the Country Women's Association where I knew no one and barely came home to sleep.

I spoke to my mother on the phone, and she was worried. There were boys there. It was a unisex accommodation. She was happier with me at the CWA, in the cloistered safety. I told her that I almost always stayed late at university and missed meals and came home hungry and broke. I told her that I was lonely and couldn't bear that place any more. I threatened that if it wasn't Raymont Lodge then it would be a share house with some people from my course, boys probably, a share house full of drugs and boys and sex. She agreed, reluctantly, and John helped me to move my few possessions to a room at the lodge.

The rooms were grouped around a communal kitchen. The girls in my cluster were friendly enough, but they were as alien to me as the girls at the CWA. I heard noises and smelled things coming out of their units that I couldn't identify. They showed each other makeup they had bought and set unfathomable rules for the collective kitchen, endless lists of things that should or should not be done. They were always on diets. Sometimes the units smelled of boiled cabbage, and some weeks there was nothing but silver Jenny Craig containers cluttering up the refrigerator. They shared diets and stories about boys and jokes about popular culture that I didn't understand. In the daytime there were soap operas on the communal television. At night there were sitcoms and the only difference as far as I could tell was the laugh track.

I would cross the central courtyard to John's wing with a cask of wine, which was against the house rules, and we hid it in the garden and skulled coffee cups of the stuff after dinner. It was an easier time. I still felt restless in the evenings and found myself spending time in a nearby park overlooking a train station, watching the commuters trudging home through the puddles of streetlights and reading the names of dead people on the memorial statue.

In the set of rooms close to John's I noticed a group of boys. They had pulled the table away from view and huddled around it. They would spend their evenings quietly, erupting into laughter before shushing each other back to quiet. They were an odd bunch, badly dressed and not seeming to care about that. A couple of them wore the trademark black stovepipe pants and pointy boots of goths, but even they were half-hearted about their costume, venturing out in flannelette shirts and T-shirts torn at the seams. One of the boys was the same age as me, but had a beard down to his midchest and a receding hairline that made him look quite grandfatherly. One night I ventured in for a closer look.

Dungeons & Dragons. They slapped the Dungeon Master screen down as soon as I entered their enclave but I had seen it. I could see it still, despite the heavy chemistry textbooks they nudged casually on top of it. Dungeons & Dragons was banned at Raymont Lodge, the magic and demons considered an affront to Christian values. It was specifically written into the rules. No closed doors if you had a visitor of the opposite sex, no alcohol, no drugs, and no Dungeons & Dragons.

The boys were pocketing their twenty-sided dice and their little metal figurines when I approached them. The boy closest to me smiled, a cheeky cherubic grin, and held out his hand to shake my own. Robert was studying information technology.

"Krissy," I introduced myself. "Drama student, but don't hold that against me. I play a ranger."

"Evan," said a red-haired, blue-eyed boy with a shy smile. "Girls don't play Dungeons & Dragons."

"Well I do, and I have wine. I think that entitles me to join your game."

I sat between Robert and Evan and filled their coffee cups under the table. We played quietly, secretly. When we heard people approaching we hid the module under textbooks and pretended to talk about exams. I laughed. It was the first time I had laughed since leaving Dragonhall. I teased the boys and they teased back and we became friends quickly. I was invited back the next night and the night after that and soon they knew how I liked my tea and sometimes Evan would wander across the complex carrying two cups of tea, spinning them in twine slings he had crocheted to prove the existence of centrifugal force, not a drop spilled. I still spent time with John but it was not just John. I had friends now, a group of them, and sometimes we wandered into the city, and sometimes we caught a train to the cinema and I would come with them to Hungry Jacks afterward to watch them eat greasy burgers, excusing myself by explaining my vegetarianism.

I bought pointy black shoes like some of the boys and listened to Bauhaus.

James made the trip down from Gladstone to visit me and although I missed the evenings playing Dungeons & Dragons, the thought of sex was more immediate. James and I touched and kissed and petted but he still refused to have sex with me. "For your own good," he said, and I never knew what he meant by that.

He left me to masturbate by myself, I shut myself in my room and drew the curtains and spent hours at it, coming and then resting and then coming again.

Then I had a dream about Evan.

I liked him. Many wouldn't, but I did. He had an awkward sense of humor. Sometimes it didn't seem like he was telling a joke, but hours later I would repeat something he'd said and find the humor in it. He talked a lot about computers, which were then new to the world. Some of us had them, huge boxy things with barely any memory. I printed my assignments out on a dot matrix printer and watched the paper catch and feed out all askew.

I still liked my typewriter with the two-line memory and the automatic corrective action that seemed to make the words vanish off the page with just the press of a key. He preferred my computer. He liked talking about old *Star Trek* episodes. He liked Mr. Spock and I liked McCoy and we agreed that explained the difference between us. Still, we were fond of each other. He made me cups of tea and didn't even ask the other gamers if they wanted one. I sometimes put a weedy flower in the keyhole of his dorm room because I knew that no one ever brought him flowers.

I dreamed that we were in the bath together playing D&D. There were other people in the room, the whole gothic, geeky, overnourished, undersunned bunch of them. All of them with their little painted figures of magic users and dwarfs and rangers. Someone was rolling the multisided die and it was skittering loudly on the tiled floor. No one seemed to mind that Evan and I were naked in the bath. No one seemed to mind when I ducked down under the water to suck on his penis, an impulse I found odd even in the dream since I had never wanted even to touch him before this. I liked him. He was fond of me. There was a kind of familial easiness between us that we appreciated, but I had never even thought about his body under his pointy boots and his black trench coat.

In the dream there were these little dives under the surface of the water. There was this held-breath suckling as if I were a child and his penis rose like a nipple in front of me. I tasted his pearly pre-come and it was sweet as milk. I would rise up for air and someone would tell me to roll the dice and I would ask them to roll it for me. A twenty-sided die, which is almost a sphere, juddering across the hard surface.

"You've been stabbed in the arm by an orc," the dream-nerd Evan told me and I shrugged, took a deep breath, and went down to nuzzle at the orange fur dusting his balls like peach fuzz.

It was a strange dream. Unexpected. I sat opposite him in the common room and we had our little metal figurines in front of us and there was the Dungeon Master's screen between us and I found myself blushing.

He stood and went out to the kitchen and came back with two

cups of tea. One for him. One for me. No one seemed to notice. This was what he always did. I was the only girl that played and I suppose he did this out of a sense of chivalry. He put the cup of tea down in front of me and smiled and I wondered if his pubic hair really was the same color as his beard.

EVAN

I had sex with Evan because I wanted a ticket to the movies. I have to be honest about this.

He won tickets to the preview of *Little Shop of Horrors*. I imagined sitting in the cinema and my nostrils filled with the scent of popcorn, a comforting chocolate Malteser kind of smell, childhood and heavy petting and Sunday afternoon all rolled into a plush red seat. I thought about that movie all through dinner. I dreamed it, fantasized the ending. I even found myself wondering about the characters during Cultural Studies. I wanted to go. I opened my wallet and counted the money there, almost enough for a bus ticket. I wanted Evan's extra ticket and so I seduced him one afternoon.

It was his first time. It crossed my mind that a virginity was probably worth more than the cost of a ticket to the movies and I felt a little guilty, but I liked him. I liked the way he shuddered nervously and became very quiet, looking up at me as if I were an angel, deflowering him in a halo of heavenly light. I liked the way he was made, the compact muscles and the strong curve of his legs. I liked the way he waited for me to show him where and how and the way he listened when I told him what to do and why to do it. I liked his studiousness, his bookishness. I liked the way he came too quickly but was quite prepared to come again before too long.

Afterward he glanced up at me briefly, gratefully. He seemed surprised to be here with me at all. And there was that shy penis, hiding in its foreskin. A strange new piece of male anatomy that I had never seen before. He shuddered when I sucked on it. He seemed to feel every small movement of my tongue. He eased my head away when I became too eager in my attentions. His tender shy penis, a pleasant surprise hiding beneath the horror show of eighties clothing.

I felt a nibble of regret. I had stuck with James for quite a while but I wanted sex, and he wouldn't give it to me and he wouldn't move to Brisbane and so that was the end of it. I settled back down onto the new thing, this D&D playing computer programmer who brought me cups of tea in his little crocheted slings, and it felt okay.

Later, in the fading afternoon, I asked him about the ticket, but he had already promised it to his friend. I watched them leave for the movies together. I stayed at home and drank tea and wondered, until they returned home gloriously happy and showed me the prize that had been hidden under their theater seat. They were best friends. I liked that he had stuck with his promise to his best friend.

That night I came into his bedroom and taught him things. He smelled a bit like chocolate, and there was a kernel of popcorn caught in the cuff of his jeans.

I longed for the cinema all through the long slow fucking. He was a nice man, quiet, and with the kind of eyes that could be cold or blazing if you caught them in a particular light. He was intelligent and had a nice body. I had flirted with him as I flirted with any of them, intermittently and without much commitment, but he was almost my favorite. I liked the short boy with curly hair who used to bang his forehead against the wall whenever his computer wasn't working, too. There was not much between them, the fire-eyed boy and the boy with mild Aspergers. It could have gone either way.

Except for that ticket to the movies.

SHARE HOUSE

When we moved out of Raymont Lodge I bought a bed. A bed and sheets. I had an image in my head of silk sheets, thick and heavy, sheets that you could wrap your naked flesh in and have pleasure just from the shrouding. The synthetic satin was a concession to my poor financial status. The sheets were cheap but they were a bright red and they looked beautiful and felt quite nice until the polyester started to sweat.

A bed was more difficult. I wanted something large, some king-size wonder of engineering. I wanted a bed you could spend months on. A virtual boat of a bed made for languid fucking, pillows like marshmallows, smelling faintly of expensive perfume.

I decided on a waterbed on someone else's recommendation and the glitz of porno-chic appealed to me. There was an excessiveness that suited. I imagined a thousand liquid nights and the delight of a back and forth rocking, a boat tied to shore but still caught by a gentle tide, tugging me toward a boundless ocean.

We filled the bed and lay down, and an icy cold caught me in the kidneys. I shivered. The thing would take twenty-four hours to warm up. I was determined to have sex on it despite this, but the positioning was impossible. If you lay on your back there was the issue of the cold. If you knelt there was the impossibility of the waves, each little thrust caught on a tide and magnified in a series of ever-larger ripples. It made us laugh and tumble over onto our sides, in which position we took to shivering. We put on sweaters, coats, socks. We made a woolly bundle of our bodies leaving peepholes in the layers through which to touch each other. We spent a joyous time experimenting with the oceanic roll of waves. There was much laughter, but at the end of it all we climbed down onto the carpet, shedding our layers of winter woollies on the way and burned our knees on the old short pile. We lay on the postcoital carpet and I dragged the satin sheets off the bed and they were too hot and made me sweat.

I woke and rolled over onto the hard ache of the space beside him and I told him about my disappointment in the sheets and the fact that I had probably spent everything I had on a king-size bed that I couldn't fuck in.

"We'll fuck on the floor."

He pulled me to him and he had the most beautiful clear blue eyes, full of a need for me to like him. I did. I lay on the floor beside my waterbed and shut my eyes tight and I hugged him and wondered if I had finally come home.

There were a few of us in the house. A motley bunch of Dungeons & Dragons players, a goth, the Asperger's boy. We all gathered at our house on weekends and pulled our little metal figures from their drawstring bags. We set up the screen and rolled the dice, but I was already tiring of the routine.

Sometimes the boys would come over to watch pornography. You could rent the hard stuff from some video stores, you just had to ask them. It was always my job to ask because the boys were too embarrassed. It made them feel like perverts. They said it was different for girls. It wouldn't look like I was dirty, I would just be liberal minded. Brave and bold and unrepressed. Still, every time I went up to the counter the man there looked me up and down and it was clear he thought I might well be a pervert; and one that he might contemplate fucking if the lights were off and he was drunk enough.

We watched the pornography in the dark because that's what you were supposed to do. We sat there with cups of tea, three of us, sometimes four. We watched and when it was over we stomped around the flat for a minute or two before slouching off to our respective bedrooms. Sometimes we snickered at the terrible attempts at comedy—the one with the fireman, the one with the doctor, the one with the tradesman and the plumbing problem.

One night someone lifted himself up from out of the couch and knelt by the video player and pressed rewind. We watched it again.

"You've got to be kidding me."

And again. But each time we watched it we saw the same thing, a man with his entire fist buried in a girl up to the elbow. She looked less than comfortable. She whimpered and grimaced and winced. Measuring the potential length of his arm, we silently calculated the position of his fist. Somewhere up near her stomach.

"How is such a thing even possible?"

In the spirit of scientific enquiry we pressed rewind and watched the video again.

I remembered the scene later, during several failed attempts at a similar scenario. "How did he even get his knuckle through in the first place?" My snickering dislodged Evan's slippery fist yet again.

We had used most of a tube of KY and he had small hands, delicately tapered fingers. I thought perhaps that we might manage it with a little persistence. We came back to the idea repeatedly. I thought about the scene from the porno. The sweaty gasps, half pain, half pleasure. I wondered if the process was damaging her in some way. The close shot showed his elbow, slick with lube, protruding from the slick mouth of her vagina. There was a little bit of movement, perhaps a centimeter, as the man braced himself against the table and put the weight of his shoulder behind the process. We didn't see the entry or what might have been the gory retreat, his limb pulled in excruciating inches from the livid mess of her. We saw his elbow pushing in and out a fraction. We saw a pained close shot of her face, teetering on the line between pleasure and regret.

If Evan's knuckles were just a little slimmer I might have some sense of what this could be like. We failed every time. The effort of it, the straining, and the image reflected back at me when he held up a little mirror, tipped me over the edge and after that I had no interest in continuing the experiment.

It was only years later, traveling across the Story Bridge, imagining what I would be cooking for a dinner party, that I realized he was an amputee. This must have been the trick to it. From a lifetime's worth of strange questions lodged in my brain and puzzled over by my subconscious, this conundrum was answered, suddenly and without provocation. He must have been an amputee. We never saw his fist enter her or retreat. All we saw was this small movement, this in and out of his elbow.

Well, we were young and naïve and, although we knew they were rare, odd things like the whole-forearm fisting scene still seemed like a possibility.

Sometimes Evan gave me things. One was perhaps the most romantic present anyone had ever given me. When I unwrapped it I found something he had made himself, put time and effort into. Some kind of battery thing that whirred and jiggled when you flicked a switch, and then gaffer tape holding the jeweled green handle of a screwdriver in place.

I wasn't certain when I first opened the wrapping. I was all, "Oh, thanks" without really understanding, until he turned it on and it started to buzz and the green end bounced quickly back and forth.

I knew about vibrators. I had seen them in porn but I had never actually met one in real life. Now I did. A homemade thing constructed with a little skill and a lot of tenderness. A little Tonya Todman perhaps, but I was pleased with it.

Evan unwrapped me in turn, and there was a click of plastic on bone when the new toy rattled against my pubis. He pressed the screwdriver end inside me and the sound of it was muffled by his hand, the various folds and clutches of flesh. I could feel the shudder of it echo out toward my skin. A little twitching, and I was quick to distance myself from the situation, talking myself down, because it would all be over if I jumped off too quickly.

My skin was twitchy tingly. I dragged his head toward me and kissed his open mouth and whispered love into him.

It was difficult to stay removed from my body, the vibrations called me back into myself. I wanted it to last, but of course it didn't and I tripped into the disappointment of an early conclusion.

RESTLESS

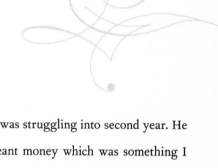

Evan finished university while I was struggling into second year. He found a good job, and a job meant money which was something I seemed to have less and less of. He went out to pubs with our friends who had also started to earn a wage. They went to movies that I could not afford. I found myself excluded from any aspect of his life that related to recreation. In the evenings he watched television with our flatmate. I could hear their laughter as I hunched over my assignments and my novel in progress. I began to look at other people. Passing strangers aroused me.

We fucked regularly, but it had become something he did to placate me. I wanted sex and therefore he roused himself from whatever else he was doing and gave me sex. The hollowness of the act echoed. "You always want sex. Sometimes it's okay not to have sex."

But it was true, I did always want sex, and sometimes I saw it everywhere. I remember one bus journey particularly. A group of schoolgirls, all giggly and blond and fine tanned skin from a bottle, their uniforms too short at the waist and the little indentations of their belly buttons marring the perfectly flat surface of their stomachs. I was barely older than them: in my early twenties, but they were teenagers as I had never been a teenager.

You could smell them, the high school smell of cheap perfume and sweat and heat. The heat was something else, I could feel it through my knees, which were closer to them. When the bus lurched and one of them fell toward my lap there was heat in there, too. I wanted them to be naked. I wanted this more than anything in that moment. I was appalled at myself, but I wanted it. They were ripe. They were peach fuzz and perfect sweet flesh. I wanted to bite down into them before the flesh was spoiled by their slow trudge toward death.

I became a monster in that moment of longing. They would look at me if they knew and curl their lips back in disgust. They would look at my flesh, which was never beautiful, and smell my damp earth muskiness and make hideous squealing noises in disgust.

I started to walk again. It would happen in the evenings, when the boys were settled down to bad American TV. I would hear them laugh as I shut the door behind me and they would barely notice I was gone. I would walk and then sometimes I would be overtaken by a wave of panic and I would run, as if something was chasing me. Sometimes I thought something was actually chasing me. Sometimes I heard it behind me and I glanced around and it was nothing but traffic.

I had felt this before. I remembered my days at the Country Women's Association and I remembered, also, a nostalgic scene in our backyard, waiting for Dragonhall to be built. I remember telling my sister about it—something is wrong. Something is terribly wrong. I don't see the point anymore. I can't find a good enough reason to keep going. I had felt this before and therefore I would feel this again, and the day-to-day of it all was not enough to keep me trudging on.

I stopped at a chemist thinking I would buy sleeping pills, but I didn't know what to ask for. I pointed to the largest packet of extra strength aspirin and paid for it with the last of my Austudy money. I half-walked, half-ran back to our home.

The boys barely glanced up from the television screen. I slunk through to the bathroom and I heard them laughing and I was invisible. I took the whole packet of tablets because I thought that might do it. I could go to sleep then and the strange sense of panic would be gone. I lay on our waterbed and it was the rocking I think, the rocking and an odd dizziness. I was up as quickly as I could struggle out of the sagging bladder of the bed and vomiting into the toilet, a little onto the floor and there were tablets in it. A scatter of half-dissolved tablets all over the tiles.

"Stupid girl."

Evan held my hair back from my face as I vomited, and he cleaned up after me. He made me drink so much water that I vomited again and even then he forced my head back and poured water down my throat.

"Stupid girl." He stroked my head on the pillow and I was terribly tired and couldn't stop crying. I remembered the CWA, and I was thinking, this will get better and then it will happen again and right now it feels like the end of the world, and even if tomorrow is a brighter day, there will be another and another, and the army of days stretching ahead made me hoist a white flag and lie back in the bed and hope that I had ingested enough tablets to ease me away from the world.

I hadn't. I woke late the next day. My eyes were finally dry and the light was too bright and my head ached so badly that I could barely think. One thought bobbed to the surface and floated there.

I just can't drift along like this. Something has to change. Something has to change.

BECOMING CATHERINE DENEUVE

Brisbane 2008

Every day I come back to my computer. I trawl through my sex life, one post at a time. I begin to find the patterns, the back and forth clacking of the ping pong ball. I have bounced between one lover and another and I remember the sex. Most of my other memories are vague, a watercolor wash of people and places I only half recall. The sex remains strikingly clear. Visceral: I remember the sex in my body. I smell it on me when I have finished a blog post and emerge, tired and a little confused back into the real world, in my aging body. Who am I now, I wonder. Where have I left myself?

My blog posts unearth a pattern. I am growing older and the fear that I might lose my sexuality to the passing of years is palpable.

We all grow up to be somebody. We make ourselves up, one

piece at a time, from all the possibilities around us. When I grow up I want to be as warm and cuddly as my mother. When I grow up I want to be as kick-ass as Batgirl. When I grow up I want to be Catherine Deneuve.

And then we grow up and we become the same person we were as a child, only with affectations gleaned from comic books and movie stars and real-life heroes. Underneath the various masks nothing much has changed.

Approaching my fortieth birthday, I look at my dirty laundry, aired publicly on my blog posts, and I know suddenly that I will not grow up to be Catherine Deneuve. I will not magically become the refined but impossibly sexy French superstar despite the hours of watching, pressing rewind, watching, longing, watching.

When I am forty I will be the same unsettled, scatty child who grew bored of climbing a tree halfway up; who could weep for the loss of a toy and, a matter of days later, not remember the toy at all. Who could turn around and start a book again from the beginning, and come to the ending as full of wonder as if I had never visited it before.

I am a middle-aged married woman. I sometimes glaze through my days in a cloud of forgetting, swept up in a hungry tide of wanting. I allow myself to wander freely amongst all of this romantic possibility forgetting that, one, I am old; two, I am not particularly attractive; three, I am married.

I am beginning to realize that when I grow up, which surely

must be any day now, there will be no satisfying turnaround where my ordinary life crashes against my fantasy realm and I finally become the real me.

Christopher invites me for a beer after work and I sit with him and I try my hardest, but I can't even conjure up a sliver of attraction toward him. I have been chatting to Paul on the Internet and now Christopher has been usurped. I don't even remember what Paul looks likes, just a vague impression, but we talk every night. I feel like his voice is my own voice, and I feel an attraction built on disembodied words.

"Do you know that boy, Paul, your writer friend? The one we met at that festival?"

Christopher nods.

"Should I invite him for a drink with us one day?"

"We can go for a drink," he tells me, but his eyes have narrowed down to a suspicious squint. "If you want to, we can go for a drink with him."

I look at Christopher now and I feel the warm glow of my fondness. I say, "You know I think we'll be friends till the day I die."

He looks at me cautiously and orders me another beer.

BREAKUP SEX

Brisbane 1989

I lay next to Evan and we were holding hands, sticky with our sweat and juices. I could hear his blood pounding through his wrist.

"Why didn't we have sex like that when we were together?" he asked, and I turned away because I was afraid I might cry.

I was there when he opened the door and not a word was spoken. We kissed, a gentle kiss with the door wide open behind us. A pause to close it, and an irresistible descent into the kind of passion that we never managed when we were together, and a lurching sensation which I realized was our love for each other surfacing briefly, bobbing up and falling away again. The corpse of it, sinking.

The sex we had that night was not the comforting kind that we had grown used to. We stole pieces off each other, samples of skin secreted away under our fingernails, the taste of sweat, the bitter burn of his semen that I would taste at the back of my throat for days. He pressed his thumb into my skin so fiercely that I felt the flesh give and his fingerprint is still on me, a lasting scar.

We didn't speak of the bad times, but they were there, too, in the way we tugged at each other's hair and in the tears that streamed from our eyes into each other's mouths.

We lay in the ruin of our relationship and the glory of our sex, all contradictions, loving each other and hating that there was nothing left to do but part.

"Why didn't we have sex like that when we were still together?"

"Because we were still together."

THE ARCHITECT

"You see," the architect explained, "you're just not the girlfriend kind."

And of course I wondered if he thought this because I had just enjoyed anal sex for the first time. Perhaps girlfriends didn't let their boyfriends slip it into their back passage. Perhaps girlfriends contrived to appear violated at the very thought, pretended to grimace in pain when their boyfriends dared to breach the sacred threshold. Despite the modest size of their boyfriend's penis.

I was sweating from the effort of it all, an energetic oral titillation with barely a hint of reciprocation. Of course I had enjoyed it. There had been days of teasing. The architect, I can't remember his name now but I'm sure it was something double-barreled, was from good stock. Moneyed. His clothes were fine and he was fond of telling me the brand name of his shirts, even though the name meant nothing to me. He did look good. He was good in bed. I had been sleeping with him for over a week and of course, given the repetition of our meetings, I thought we might have graduated from casual acquaintance to something in the realm of dating.

"Don't take offense," he told me, struggling with the knot in the top of his condom, dabbing himself clean with a tissue.

I would have hated him at that moment, but the sex had been good and I wanted to like him enough to do it again. This was the first sex I had had since the breakup, and it felt good to be touched again, good to escape the neat suburban haven of my temporary flatmates.

"But there's this girl I met and she's more like a girlfriend type, if you know what I mean."

I didn't.

"You're sexy," kisses then and nuzzling and really, I didn't like him all that much, but the thought that I was something less than the girlfriend type seemed to itch at me. I wanted this boy, the architect, this spoiled little rich kid with his designer shirts, to like me more than he liked her.

"She's a nurse."

I could be a nurse.

"At the hospital."

I could dress in a little white dress with nice sensible white shoes. I could wear good underwear beneath it; no underwear, perhaps. I was sure he would like it if I turned up, pantyless with a sponge bath.

"You met her . . . ?"

"On Saturday. At a party."

Saturday was three days, half a relationship, ago. The real girlfriend settling into place quietly in the background and him, the architect, tickling my asshole with his fingertip, counting the days in subtle coercions. Just a fingertip, then the whole finger, then here, on day three, a full-scale anal penetration before beating a hasty retreat.

"Come on. Don't be like that. Surely you know you're not the girlfriend type."

I knew it. Even then, when it was only him, the appalling architect, informing me of my shortcomings. I knew it. There was something unusual about my passion for sex. I consumed it as real girlfriends might consume chocolates, licking their fingers afterward, savoring the smell of it on their breath. Three other men would tell me later that I was not a "girlfriend" kind of girl. A repetition of a theme. One of these men was kind enough to pick out friends of mine as examples—her, she's a girlfriend kind, and her. A considerate lover.

I was not the girlfriend kind, but he shrugged when I asked if I would meet him tomorrow.

"So long as you know," he told me. "So long as you don't get attached."

But the blindfold may have been one step too far. He was up for it, of course. He knew I would take him somewhere secret. He let me tie the cloth around his face, inching his crotch toward me, eager to begin the night's proceedings.

I had arranged a driver, Lucy, a friend of mine.

My architect hadn't expected Lucy to be there either. As he heard her voice, a whispered call to action, I felt him shrink. But by this time I had tied his arms behind his back, tightly enough to make it difficult for him to escape. She was good with knots. She had shown me how to tie the rope, and it worked. I grinned at her and pulled hard enough to make him flinch.

I was new to this. Until now it had all been one more petal pulled off a fragile flower. He loves me or he doesn't, the flowers all tacked together like a daisy chain. I looked back on my insipid handful of lovers and they were all smudged over as if they had been shot in soft focus with Vaseline smeared on the lens. They were David Hamilton photographs, and me in my billowing black dress, running through some field or other.

I tied his hands and he was shaking, only partly with pleasure. He barely knew me and he was putting himself at my mercy. His edginess made me feel warm, a little inflated with possibilities that I had never even considered before this.

I took him to the mountains.

He tried to speak in the car and I told him not to. I told him that he should just listen to the sound of the tires on gravel, the sound of the sealed roads slipping away. Smell the pungent scents of the country edging in through the windows.

I laid him on an unfamiliar bed in an unfamiliar house. I left the blindfold on him, left his hands tied. I undressed him and found there was no way to take his shirt off without releasing his hands. I could have ripped it. They do that kind of thing in movies and in books. I could have found the scissors and cut the fabric at a seam. It would have added to it all, the sound of the scissors snipping through the expensive linen, but I could never save up enough out of my Austudy to replace it, so I left him with his shirt unbuttoned. I licked his chest, found the rising buds of his nipples and sucked on them, one at a time.

I moved lower, concentrating on the straining penis, just enough spit to lubricate the inside of the condom. I was going to concentrate on my own pleasure. This was something that I had never done with a partner before.

I stood and watched his body unobserved. It was a fine collection of skin and muscle and bone, a strong body, thin but well formed. I watched it, but there was no quick lurch of desire in my stomach at the sight of his erection. When I turned him over on the bed I saw the tight curve of his ass and it was fine and quite beautiful but I felt no emotional attachment to the thing. I touched it. I settled myself on top of it, straddling the curve of flesh. I traced the indentation with my thumbs. He bucked back against me. He wanted me inside him. This was something we had done before, something I enjoyed, but his insistence turned me off the whole idea.

I lifted myself off him and went to my overnight bag. My vibrator was a small finger of black plastic. Nothing special, just one speed, a minimum of fuss. Tonight I would focus on my own pleasure. Just me, my vibrator and the blind body of this other person.

I would take my pleasure.

He wriggled in frustration, a landed fish. There was, of course, the quick image of a short knife gutting. In my new role as aggressor, I felt an underlying possibility of violence simmering. Something shifted between us.

I lowered myself onto him and I would be lying if I said I didn't enjoy the power of it.

Finally, a few days later, he gave me the handgrip from a bicycle and settled against the wall. He wanted to watch. I suppose I knew that this would be the last time for us. There was no kiss hello, no hug, just a handing over of the implement.

"I want to watch," he said and settled, just like that.

"You want me to masturbate?"

"Yes."

"You want to watch?"

"Yes."

I could have said no I suppose, but this was an adventure I had never been on. I was always up for an adventure.

"Open them." Like the disembodied voice intruding on a scene from a pornographic movie. "Now spit."

I glared. As if the boy could direct me toward orgasm better than I could direct myself.

"Be quiet," I told him. "Or I won't be able to come."

"I don't care if you come or not."

And so the line was drawn. I raced him, from my position perched on the edge of his bed. I watched him, fully clothed but for the ridiculous protrusion of his penis, his hand on it. No spit for him. He had the bottle of lubricant and he used it liberally. I would make this about me, I thought, about my orgasm. I could use him just as well as he would use me. I watched him stroke himself in that halting, a-rhythmic way he had and I wanted to get off on it, but I found myself hating him instead. A little bit more with every stroke.

He directed me from his lazy lean, removed from the activity yet involved. When he was close the directions stopped. He closed his eyes and I watched his whole body tense and I watched him catch his ejaculate in the palm of his hand.

I sat on the edge of the bed with the handle from a bicycle inside me and I didn't want to continue. We would not continue. He wiped his hand on a tissue and zipped himself up and he looked unruffled.

"Thanks for that."

When he walked out into the lounge room to get a beer I knew that I would never see him again and that was okay, too. I didn't particularly like him with his nice clothes and his fetish for nurses. I liked the sex, which was always detached and slightly angry, but I didn't like waking up beside him and I had rarely slept over for this reason.

He was expecting me to stay for a beer, but I gathered up my things and I left. I left the bicycle handle on his clean black bedspread where it would drip and stain and he would have to wash the whole thing, which would annoy him.

MEETING IN REAL LIFE

Brisbane 2008

Christopher is looking out for Paul because he knows him better, but I remember Paul as soon as I see him. I wasn't sure I would. Christopher and I have chatted our way through two beers and then Paul is here, suddenly, and I know it is him. He has a manner which is both confident and shy at the same time, as if he is apologizing for his own self-assurance. I recognize his voice. He never wavers in his manner. It is the same rhythm and meter that I enjoy so much from our electronic chatting. There is comedic timing, and Paul is quick. He leaps from one topic to another like a dancer. He can take us both, Christopher and I, engaging with our similarities and our differences.

I buy him a beer.

We turn our attention to people we have in common. This is

one of those towns where people wash up against each other. Huddles of people bob on a cyclical Brisbane tide. I have probably slept with friends of his mother's or at least friends of her friends. It is inevitable. We find people in common and we circle around them.

Paul likes girls, it seems. Girls like him. Girls that I have had altercations with like him. He likes some girls who dislike me and actively make my life difficult. He mentions their names and extols their virtues. He likes them and he will not back down. My glower is a siren, warning him against shallow water and sharp rocks. Paul is perhaps a little drunk and therefore unable to read me neatly. He blusters on.

I am becoming irritable as I down another glass of wine. "We should stop talking about her, maybe."

Christopher suggests a meal. He is more sensitive to my moods than Paul, it seems. He wants us up and walking. We move to a restaurant nearby and it seems the fresh air has lightened things. We talk about food, swap recipes. Paul likes to cook and I have a knack with herbs and spices. It seems our ship has righted itself. I push off into safer waters and he sails alongside me, but in a pause he mentions another girl, my arch-nemesis. He counts the things he likes about her, her manner, her habit of giggling and touching him on the arm. I tell him that this is an affectation, that I would never use such calculated moves to charm someone, but Paul will not budge from his admiration and when our food arrives, I eat it with a tight throat. At one point I think I might choke on a chicken burrito, but I swallow it and chase it down with more wine.

The problem with the Internet is that it is so easy both to misinterpret and to misrepresent. In the harsh light of the real world, I take stock of Paul and know that my assessment was misguided. He is an irritant. He is a charming liar. He is a clever salesman with the gift of the gab and a penchant for flirtation. I will not be flirted with by him.

When we come to the subject of dating I explain that I have never gone on dates, just one, a disaster that ended in bad sex and subsequent avoidance tactics. He says he would like to take me on a date, but at this moment that is the last thing I would want to do. I want to finish my meal, scull the last of my wine, and find the quickest path away from him. Later, I will not talk with him on the Internet. I will not be fooled by his faux-sensitive banter. He is all lies.

But still there is something about the quiet hurt in the droop of his girlish mouth and the odd style of his dress, and the slightly mannered way he speaks. Something about all of this makes me think that there must be more to him than that. Some softer place that he is hiding beneath a calculated exterior.

CAUTIONARY TALES

Brisbane 1989

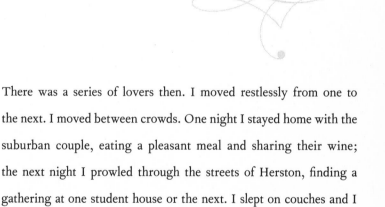

There was a series of lovers then. I moved restlessly from one to the next. I moved between crowds. One night I stayed home with the suburban couple, eating a pleasant meal and sharing their wine; the next night I prowled through the streets of Herston, finding a gathering at one student house or the next. I slept on couches and I stayed awake in bars until late. There was very little money, but I could walk vast distances, I had practiced. I could wander from one place to the other. There was university and then I found a sign for café staff needed and got the job. There was a little more money then and I could prowl the late night bars for potential partners.

I played, but I played in relative safety. Condoms were essential, bareback was not an option. These were the days of the grim reaper ads and I knew I could die from it.

There exists a kind of dating etiquette, I realized, that I had never learned. I developed my own code of honor through trial and error. I would say no to anyone who approached me unless they seemed nervous and unpracticed. I would approach a potential lover on my own terms and with no encumbrances. I would not accept free drinks: I was not repaying drinks with favors, I was making a conscious choice. And I rarely went back to their house, choosing to consummate in a side street or at a friend's house or my own.

There were, of course, experiences along the way that led to the getting of this wisdom.

1. Paying Your Own Way

I had to sleep with him because he paid for dinner. Not just dinner but drinks as well. I tried to pull my wallet out but he waved it aside and I felt my enthusiasm dissipate. Now I would have to sleep with him and I had had to endure his conversation for a whole evening, a boy who never seemed to tire of talking about himself.

This was my first actual date, when someone asked me out and not the other way around, and I realized then why I had never dated. It was the conversation, scraping at the fabric of a perfectly fine evening with the fingernail shriek of his voice.

The pillowcase was an inspiration. The imperative was to find a way to stop him kissing me. He had a nagging tongue that kept invading my mouth, a hard probing tongue. It made me think of the dentist's chair and I couldn't breathe because of it. I wanted to spit it out. I'm not sure why I thought of the pillowcase, but suddenly it was there and I reached for it and jammed it over his head, a kind of cotton bag that kept his tongue away from the inside of my cheeks. He still kissed me through the yellowed fabric, but it was a chaste kiss, inoffensive, and with his face hidden he could have been anyone. I imagined that he was someone else, someone who hadn't bored me for the better part of the evening, someone who hadn't paid for my dinner at an expensive restaurant.

Even with the bag, I could hear him, droning on and on, sex talk. How could sex talk be so monotonous?

The stocking was a masterstroke. I tied it around his chattering mouth and he became silent all of a sudden. Another stocking for his hands and he could not even squeeze and poke at me. I felt myself relaxing into the anonymity of the event. When he groaned I shushed him and he quietened miraculously. I began to enjoy the blank canvas of his body. I fished my vibrator out from under the pillow and let him buck his hips up to meet my strokes, one small compensation and it seemed to make all the difference to him. He came as quickly as I did and as silently.

He called. He called and called and called. I told my roommate I was out, and he relayed the information into the receiver—"She says she's out"—making me laugh. You could probably hear it over the phone.

My roommate asked me why I was avoiding the man and I told him and he could barely understand. "But you slept with him," he said, incredulous. "You tied him up and gagged him and slept with him. He must think all his Christmases have come at once. Why did you do that if you hated him?"

"He paid for dinner," I told him. "And drinks."

I don't think he ever understood my reasons, but he kept fending off the poor boy's calls as a true friend must.

"I'd sleep with you, too, if you were bagged and gagged," I teased, but the truth is I would have slept with him butt naked in the bright moonlight without blinking. I was fond of him and he was fond of me, but when I suggested it, he shook his head.

"You're just not my type, my love," he said.

2. Excessive Alcohol Consumption

And then he fell asleep. Rolled onto his back and fell asleep. Just like that.

". . . rolled onto his back and fell asleep."

"What? Just like that?" said my roommate.

"Just like that."

I shouldn't have said anything, of course. The situation brought my sexual prowess into question and I was quite proud of my prowess. I wrapped the duvet around me tightly and sat at the kitchen table, and he settled a cup of tea in front of me. The comfort of steam. I sniffed.

"He was fine when he was on top, it's just when we changed places. He just seemed to close his eyes and then . . . that was it."

"Fell asleep . . ."

"Just like that."

The man asleep in my bed would be shivering through his dreams, since I had left him nothing but a cotton sheet to keep the night away. I huddled into the warm layers of my quilt and held the fragrant cup against my lower lip.

"Am I boring? Do you find me boring?"

"Of course not. He had too much to drink."

"I'm going to tell him about it in the morning."

"I know you are."

"I will."

"I know it."

I sipped. He'd turned over onto his back and I was on top and I was just finding a rhythm when I looked down and saw that he had fallen asleep.

"Just like that. I can't believe it."

And he tutted like the good friend he was and sipped his tea.

3. Letting Them Sleep Over

Dark night of the soul and no sleep anywhere but in the slack face of this strange lover. Flaccid penis, hair sweating into my pillow. Dead to my pacing and the wringing of my hands.

Sex like a drug buzzing in my bloodstream. I'd been calmed by the orgasm, the chemical release of pheromones, but after the lull I was all wound up again. I was awake and pacing and I would run out into the dead night, the hot night teeming with the little scuttering of cockroaches, the insect hum of traffic lights. I was held to this prison of my own bedroom by a sleeping stranger who might wake to an empty house.

What if he did? If he woke and I was gone? Would he leave? Would he take something of mine with him? What was mine to take? I had nothing of great value, an armful of photographs torn from magazines, some notebooks with words more precious to me than jewels, some paperbacks, scuffed with love, the pages all turned down and underlined.

The boy would wake in an empty apartment and he would think badly of me. Odd predatory girl, a house full of twigs and fairy lights, the frightening intensity of the lovemaking, the strange postcoital pacing. All wound up.

I knew that I should wake him and make good use of him, another shot of my drug, another round of mouths and fingers and genitals.

I read somewhere that nymphomaniacs are obsessed by sex because they cannot achieve orgasm. This was not my problem. My problem was the space between orgasms, the terrible chasm of daily life, the social imperatives, the pointless living. I pressed my face against the window and looked out at all that wakeful night. A thousand places to run off into.

"Soon," I whispered into the balm of dark. "I will not bring strangers home tomorrow night. Tomorrow night I will escape and race through the electric buzz of the sleeping city in peace."

4. Misdirected Emotions

I knew where Geoffrey was at every minute. At least I thought I did. I would look up from my vodka or my coffee or whatever and think, he will be riding home from the city, or, he will be listening to that band he likes in the Valley.

Sometimes I'd test myself on it and turn up at the place he would be. He was always there. I had a kind of sixth sense for him. I knew it was creepy to be hooked into his every movement as if I'd inserted a tracking device when we were having sex, but there was nothing to be done. I was plugged into him. My radar was always poised and waiting for some weird signal to arrive.

I thought that Geoffrey was me. We were similar in many ways. We were both playful as monkeys, food fights, chases, games of backgammon, some of which ended in strange illegal moves that left us breathless with laughter. We were odd, awkward in company, prone to leaving a room in a sudden panic for no reason. We were both a little mad, we made nests in other people's houses but we never seemed to settle anywhere ourselves. I once threw all his clothes out of the window of a third-story apartment, and then he threw all mine, and then we were naked in the night, daring each other to run off into the park.

I loved him, but he didn't love me. He said he would love a girl who was homely and smelled of bread dough and cake. He wanted a girl who hung her clothes up on hangers, a girl who ironed and who didn't put up with any of his nonsense. He told me this when we were in bed together and he wasn't the first one to mention my lack of feminine wiles and so I shrugged and kept at it, hoping that the delirium we shared in bed would make up for my lack of skills in the ironing department.

We fucked so hard that we tore the sheets off the bed.

"I'd love a girl who knows how to make hospital corners," he said.

5. No Spitting on a First Date

I would look up at this new person, this naked body with its curious smells, scars in unexpected places, hair or hairlessness; perhaps a stray tattoo emerging from its hiding place, a pleasant surprise. This body was a history, a childhood, a teenage angst, this was the lover of strangers and someone's child, awkward and perhaps trembling and maybe a little suspicious of the casual way I had picked him off the street and brought him to my home.

There was the dance of fingers, tongues, the threat of teeth on skin. There was the touching of this strange new body, watching the gentle rise of a penis that had not yet divulged the whole of its story.

I would be on my knees eventually at any rate. When all the

teasing had been teased out there was always oral sex. My mouth would be full and it relieved me of the pressure to speak. I had almost always said too much already. I had used words that seemed obvious, words like "cock" and "fuck" and "cunt," but when I said those words his eyes would widen and I knew that maybe I had overstepped the invisible line once again.

He would never be as confident in sex as I was. Not the boys I liked, the fine examples of geekdom, the loners and the crazed and the sad young men. They warned me with a small pressure of their hands, the model of politeness, that I should pull away now. I would need to make a choice. I knew when it was close anyway because of the salty slipperiness on my tongue. Not an unpleasant taste but one that gave me pause. I would pause. I would take breath. I would need to pull away or be prepared to swallow when the moment came.

This was a first date—it was almost always a first date—therefore I would swallow. It seemed impolite to spit on a first date. And there would be no mess to clean, no tissues; with any luck he would not want to kiss me when I had finished, which would save me from the more invasive intimacy of his tongue against mine.

There would be space afterward for me to please myself. There would be a moment of rest in which he would be dazed and slow and happy and in this space I could play unhindered, finding other parts of his body to rub against, taking what I needed without the distractions of his inexperience.

PILLION
Brisbane 2008

Paul and those girls. Just a handful of them, but enough for me to think that we could not be friends. Last night, I felt myself closing off, an irritable stepping away. But we are participating in a workshop together this morning and I said that I would give Paul a lift. So here I am right on time.

My motorcycle is high at the pillion and he has to climb up, tugging at my shoulder, but when he is seated there is a pleasant pressure of his thighs around me and he holds me gently. There have been pillions who have hugged so tight I couldn't breathe or lean into a corner. There have been pillions who are taller and bigger and shift the balance subtly but unpleasantly. Paul touches me on the waist, but without pressure. His weight settles the bike more steadily on the road.

I once said that if my bike likes my pillion then I will like them, too—like someone with a beloved dog who helps them make informed decisions about their friends. A good pillion will be a solid friend. But perhaps it has nothing to do with friendship, because last night I felt the pricking of anger and I have decided that after this trip I will not waste my time on someone who is friends with the only three people in the world that I have difficulty liking.

It is Paul's first time on a bike and I feel him tense as we pull away from the curb. The first stretch is always the most difficult and he settles quickly. When we speed up for the highway I think about how sexual the whole thing is, the reality of sitting behind someone, gripping their ass with your thighs, the trust that is involved in the whole process of riding pillion. I find myself softening to him.

We have barely been going fifteen minutes before there is a spotting on my helmet. It is going to rain. There is nothing to do but sit and let it soak through us: riding into it there is no way to keep it out. It gets in. Even with wet weather gear, which I have not brought, it gets in through your gloves, into your boots, trousers damp and sticking to your knees. I can feel twin rivulets of rain over my chest, finding a circuitous route around the swell of my breasts, puddling in my panties, a cold finger of water teasing me toward thoughts of sex. Paul will be getting wet. He will be cursing, he could be warm and dry inside a car.

His hands are on my hips. The warmth of his fingers burns

against the chill of the rain. Despite the fact that I am still irritated with him, I feel his legs rub against mine on every bump, I imagine his hands sliding forward and I am ready for this possibility if it happens. I remember the nice clean smell of him over drinks, the musky body heat. Some people are just like that, sweating out their sexuality for the world to smell.

I know that if we stopped now I could turn around and taste him, lapping sweat and rain from his skin. I know the wetness isn't just from the rain pooling in my lap. I so rarely become damp with desire, but I feel the little flutter low in my groin. The rain, the vibrations from the engine, the open road, and the memory of the smell of him.

At some point I realize we are lost.

RICHARD

Brisbane 1989

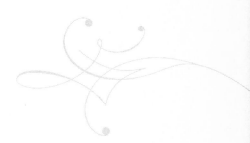

I'm not sure I would have gone out with Richard if he had been straight.

I knew he was gay and that made me look at him twice. He was sweet, thin in that helpless way I like. Hips like a girl, cute in an awkward, beaky manner. And then there was his history, the magic of all the men he had loved before me. The secret slideshow of them flicked past in my imagination, a pornographic film with this boy as the star of every frame.

This boy could be my boy. He liked me. He didn't like girls but he liked this odd girl-boy who seemed to like sex as much as he did, if not more. We could become a team. A wonderful sexy team.

I made love to his previous indiscretions. There were other men in the room with us. I imagined them all into existence. I introduced myself to them while I was in bed with him. I turned him over and I became them, telling Richard's stories back to him as he rolled onto his stomach and closed his eyes. I inhabited the young boy who lived upstairs. I lifted Richard's hips with the boy's hands and reached for the lube and I entered him with slow fingers, prizing him apart and finding a cruel rhythm just as the boy upstairs had done. I felt the power of it, the joy of being completely in control. I liked the stillness of his body beneath me.

"I want to watch you make love to a man," I told him, and he was in no position to refuse.

It was easy. I found the first man in the café. I served him coffee and he stayed and made notes in a paperback that he bent back, cracking the spine. He had been there for an hour.

"Another coffee?"

He nodded. I wasn't sure that he did want another coffee, but he wanted some more time with his cracked book and his blue pen and his furrowed brow. I chose the music for him. He had a Cure T-shirt on and I put the Cure on the stereo and watched his head nod in time to the rhythm of it.

I brought him a coffee and perched on the stool next to him. "You got much left to do?" I nodded to his book.

"Maybe half an hour. Not so long."

"I'm off work in forty minutes," I told him. "Perfect timing."

"Yes." He sat back and looked at me and I wondered what he would be seeing. A short girl, round, not particularly attractive.

Still.

"I live with a gay man," I said. "We share partners. No strings, just sex. I'm thinking we should sleep with you this evening."

I could see him struggling to find a response.

"Do whatever it is you're doing. Drink your coffee. If you decide against it you can just walk out in half an hour and we'll probably never see each other again. If you want to stay, then stay. Easy as that." I went back to the dishwasher and the food preparation and the endless table servicing.

I noticed him struggling with his reading. At some point he stopped trying. He put his pen down and closed the book and smoothed its cover. I saw that it was something by Dostoyevsky. I wondered what he was studying, but I wouldn't ask him. I didn't want to ask him. I didn't want to know his name.

He told me anyway. David. He told me as I was walking past him with two cappuccinos balanced in my hands.

"I finish in five," I told him. "And my name is Krissy."

A name wasn't anything really. I could call myself anything I wanted. I could be anyone. We caught a bus to my house and we barely said a word.

"Do you do this sort of thing often?" he asked me then.

"We will," I told him.

This was our first time and I thought it should be special, but it was nothing really. It was sex. It was fun. I liked watching Richard kiss him. I liked watching more than participating. Still, we were in this together and I let him touch me wherever he wanted and enter me wherever he wanted. I didn't orgasm, but I did later when he had left and it was just me and Richard replaying the scene from beginning to end. I kissed Richard. I came with him. I came remembering Richard's mouth on the boy's penis.

"Swallow him," I said.

"Yes, I'll suck him dry."

And then I came and it was good. Better than good. It was the kind of feeling that tingles in your limbs for the longest time.

When it had faded we rolled toward each other and hugged, and I felt safe and satisfied and alive for the first time in so very long.

"I think I love you," I told him.

And that made him cry.

PILLION 2

Brisbane 2008

We take the wrong exit off the freeway. We end up amongst the shopping centers and the run-down fish and chip shops. I smell burning fat and damp and rubber. Paul slips off the bike and he is wet, but grinning.

"I was so nervous when we started out," he says, "but then it got better."

"It is wet," I tell him, "wet and cold."

Paul nods, sniffs as if testing for the smell of rain. "Ah well, we're almost there."

But are we? We ask at a service station but the directions are complex and I am unsure.

"No, I'll remember them," says Paul.

"Okay, but tap me when we need to turn. Tap me on the right side to turn right and the left to go left."

It seems simple enough, but there are taps to both shoulders simultaneously. There are taps to the center of my back. Paul yells directions at my helmet, as if I could hear what he is saying. When we leave a side road and rattle up a horror of slippery wet grass and loose gravel I am cranky with him yet again. I do not care how good he smells and how my body wants to roll him into the mud and nuzzle into his flesh. For once my anger is more true and clear than my sexual urges; but at least we have arrived where we are supposed to be. I leave him to struggle out of his helmet and his gloves while I drag my soaking clothing up to the front door.

There is a quick tour of the house, the gorgeous excesses of each room, the bookshelves with their familiar paperbacks, books that make me feel accepted and at home. And there is a spa.

We settle in the lounge, a group of us. I perhaps have more in common with the others, middle-aged women like myself, and yet the fact that Paul and I are both dripping wet seems to mark us as similar. The others talk about the difficulties of parenting, schools, motherhood, childbirth. I sit beside Paul and he draws me into a conversation about the structuring of documentary films.

I sip my wine and I keep thinking about that spa bath, big enough for two, perhaps even three. I would not even have to remove my bra and panties. Our clothes are wet already, we could sit there fully dressed and discuss the difference between a short story writer and a novelist, whilst sipping the good wine.

The rain grows heavier. There is talk of sleeping the night. I would sleep the night. I don't want to ride home in this weather. They ask Paul what he wants to do and he pauses, looks toward me. I shrug. I could stay the night. I think about the spa bath. I try not to, but I think about the spa bath.

We could stay.

THE PRIZE

Brisbane 1989

It was all about the sex, and the sex was always fine. There was a lot of it. I was constantly buoyed along in the afterglow of one orgasm or another. I walked in a fog of sex. I was distracted by it. I bumped into things. There were always bruises. I looked at everyone as a potential partner and it was right to feel this way. Finally my world had caught up to me. I no longer felt like a secret predator, hiding my lust behind a friendly façade. I felt more honest like this. I flirted with intent. I reeled the bodies in and played with them and set them free unharmed.

On this occasion, it was all about the timing. I was at the Ryan Street house, our house, clothed in evening wear. High boots and a dress that billowed. There was opera on the stereo. All this because I couldn't bear the idea of washing up, a job I hated and rarely completed without the theater of the dress and the music. I made a performance of it, treating myself to sips of chilled wine between each burnt-bottomed pan.

When he arrived the last of the dishes was dripping foam into the precarious pile by the sink. The door was open and he stood in the lounge room and the muslin cloth was flapping in a hot breeze and I turned around and it was like a scene from some movie. Him so beautiful, me in my evening gown and my rubber gloves, the opera screaming to an exquisite climax.

I almost laughed, the poetry of the moment struck me as comical. I had given him my address but I didn't expect he would find me. He was a customer at the café and every time I spotted him perched on one of the cane stools I became inept. I dropped cups, fumbled cakes off their plates; once I even dropped a whole tray, hot with dishes just washed.

So I didn't try to speak to him when he stood in my lounge room. I took my clothes off, standing in boots and bra as the opera quietened to a duet.

I walked past him into the bedroom where our king-size futon kissed three of the walls and when he stumbled out of his trousers I noticed that his penis was too large. He was a tall man, and I was short enough to approach it warily. I could only fit a fraction of it in my mouth. I rolled the condom part of the way using my lips, but I was forced to back off, finish the job with my fingers. It was the first time this had happened to me. I wondered if it would hurt.

I was wet, which was unusual. I am not the kind of girl you read about in pornographic magazines, oozing juices. My excitement leaves me perhaps a little damp. Even after orgasm there is no more than a discreet slick, just enough to give a slippery edge. I like the feel of lubricant and face cream and spit, but I am like a desert, hot and fierce with passion but with only a hazy glimpse of moisture, a mirage.

On this day, perhaps because of the heat or the opera or the hours standing at the sink in high heels, there was little need for lubricant. I used it anyway, the size of his penis made a little knot in my lower abdomen. Too big for me. I thought he might hurt. I squeezed the clear stickiness onto my palm and marveled at the distance traveled by my fist, each stroke a journey all the way from the tip to the flat of his belly which was surprisingly pale and soft, like something newborn and desperate for protection.

I lay him on our bed, this man that I had wanted for so many weeks. I straddled his hips and settled myself down gently, only a small way.

How could I take much more of him into me? I measured the uncharted territory with my hand. I would need both hands to cover it. I stroked the vulnerable length with my fingers, my hand an extension of my cunt, massaging all the length of him. With my other arm steadying myself I wondered how I would bring myself to orgasm without loosing my grip on him completely.

The door was still open and there was Richard, standing in

the doorway, grinning. I had brought him a prize, hunter-gatherer. It could have been anyone, a stranger on a bus, someone I met at work last night, anyone. He wasn't to know that the soft groans from beneath me were the sweet chinking sounds of a jackpot paying out, the one I had wanted for so long.

He joined us without introduction. His hand linking fingers with, then replacing, my own on the generous length of penis, my body impaled on top of it, slowly relaxing to consume more of it. I felt his fingers edging into me, stretching the flexible skin, thickening the load. I felt him reach up inside me with his spidery hand and measure the length to the tip of the cock, marveling (I assumed) at the size and shape of it.

Then the fingers withdrew and I felt his tongue lapping around the boy, touching my clitoris briefly before making the long journey down to that tender pale flesh of the man's belly. I kissed the boy. He had a sensual mouth, wide and warm. His spit tasted of oranges. His tongue was long and it pushed up between my teeth and the soft underside of my lips. I wasn't sure if he had felt Richard's arrival, if he knew that the soft squeezing pressure was not some internal muscular sex-worker's trick, but the excited fingers of my lover. I had told him about Richard of course, warned him. If you find me at this address you will find Richard there as well. I kissed this new-found prize and there was a gentle pressure on my anus, a tentative testing with a fingertip followed by the cold nozzle of the lubricant and a sudden icy trickle shooting inside me, slipping around the edges, readying me for the next part of this strange dance.

It is easy to disappear when there are two penises entering you. This is what I liked most about the double entry. As long as the smaller one is in the back there is barely any physical discomfort. It is easy to become a conduit, bringing the two men together, feeling them touch through the delicate internal membrane.

There was no pressure for me to perform. The men performed for each other. I was free to watch them find each other's mouths over the slight obstruction of my shoulder. When their tongues lapped, I was there to watch. I joined the kiss only so that my tongue could see like a snail's probing feeler, sticky eye. I saw them exploring the wet cavities of each other's mouths. I felt their cocks butt up against each other. I felt them change their rhythm so that their thrusting would be synchronized.

They sucked my breasts, each tongue eager to prove itself more ardent. It was a competitive consumption of my body, their wrestling for position was half in earnest.

Richard was triumphant in the battle because he was, as always, privileged to have my anus. The grip was tighter. The position was dripping with fascination for the other lover, who was forced to content himself with a more conventional entry. I felt the new lover reach around with his extraordinarily long arm just to check that Richard really was fucking my ass. I felt him stroke the sensitive muscle with his fingertips, slipping on lubricant, forming a perfect O around Richard's penis. The extra pressure was too much for Richard. We felt the pulsing start, the two of us, this new lover and myself. We felt the uncontrollable spasms of his hips as he relinquished any thought of gentleness and pumped hard, forcing himself into me in a jerking rhythm.

The new lover thrust his head backward to expose his throat. He was about to come, too. I tried to lift myself off him to attempt a subtle retreat, but Richard was still collapsed on my back, his hips twitching in an echo of his orgasm. The boy bucked forward and it hurt, but it was also, surprisingly, pleasurable. He thrust high and hard against the shrinking swell of Richard's penis. I was flushed with the effort of taking him in. I felt the pumping of it stretching me and I pressed my thumb against my clitoris, scratched it back and forth. I wanted to come. When there was a new lover in my bed I never came. I would save it up for later when Richard and I could be alone and have more time to reflect. But this was my prize, the boy who made me spill milk, drop cups, fumble cakes into customers' laps. This was that boy and he was hurting me in his uncontrollable pleasure and I climbed with him. Richard was still inside me and the contracting must have hurt him, too, because he winced, eased himself away.

When we were done he held the base of our lover's penis, keeping the condom on while he withdrew. He peeled it off the man and felt the length of him all slippery with sperm. He slipped his lips over the head and tasted. This was against the rules of course, but I watched him do it, felt the prickle of arousal begin anew. We could go again, the three of us. The possibility was in the air. We licked the taste of each other off our skin, gently. There was time. It was barely dark. There would be time for tea or wine, or perhaps some conversation. Although when I saw their mouths meet, teeth clinking awkwardly off each other, sharing the taste of our lover's sperm, I felt my stomach lurch and I was not so sure that there would be time enough for chatter.

LAURA

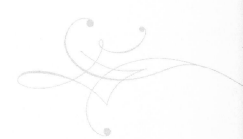

Laura, like all the girls I worked with, was beautiful. They were hired for their blond hair and their beautiful figures. They were the honey for the customers and the customers came and sipped polite little glances over their macchiatos. Some afternoons when Laura played Nina Simone on the stereo she would clamber up onto the table and dance. She wore short skirts which she made from her own patterns and plunging necklines, and her breasts were about the best I had ever seen. When I told her how much I liked them she took both my hands in her own and pushed them onto her chest.

"Feel them," she said and I did. "Feel how hard and firm they are. My mother is sixty and she still has breasts like this. I get them from my mother."

I felt her breasts and her skin was so pale and beautiful and her hair fell like silk threads long to the bottom of her skirt. She brushed it on her breaks and I could feel how wonderfully soft it was before she rolled it up and pinned it in a flirty little bun on the top of her head. She had strong hands and strong legs and she was as short as I was, but tiny, with a waist that I could almost encircle in my hands.

I didn't like to be touched, but she walked straight up to me and stroked my shoulders and rubbed my neck and I found I liked it. She smelled sweet, like honeysuckle, and had an abrupt honesty that reminded me of me.

"I like black men," she said one day when the Somalian man had stood at the counter chatting over a short black. "I like their cocks. Big fat uncut cocks."

I told her about Richard and she laughed and said that it sounded like a beautiful relationship.

"How do you do anal sex?" she asked. "I've tried but it hurts too much."

"Well you don't do it with fat uncut cocks," I explained.

We became friends.

"Will we ever sleep together?" I asked her one day when the shop was empty.

"I don't know. Do you sleep with girls?"

"I haven't, but I'd like to."

"I think I'm heterosexual."

"I don't believe in that stuff. We are just sexual, not one thing or another, just a preference, not a definite line."

"Well, I prefer boys."

If we slept together we might fight. But I liked her, and I liked her body. When she invited me back to her place, she took all her clothes off and plunged naked into the pool. When I joined her she hugged me, lifting her legs, wrapping them around my waist, pressing her perfect breasts against my own, which seemed saggy in comparison. She compared our bodies without any hint of shyness. She pointed to her pink nipples and my brown ones. She held her pale and lightly freckled skin up to my sallow flesh, so oily and brown when I sat in the sun for any length of time. I found that it was enough just to touch her. She opened her thighs to me and made me shave her pubic hair and I touched her labia.

"I get so wet. Feel that," and slipped my finger inside along with her own.

I masturbated, dreaming of her labia or her breasts or her hair, but it was never the whole person. I loved her too much to break whatever special thing had grown between us. She was always chasing after one boy or another and we shared our stories and touched and experimented with drugs occasionally but without much commitment.

She watched me leave work with one man after another.

"I admire the way you can do that," she said to me one day.

"What?"

"Just have sex for the sake of it. I always have to invent some kind of undying love."

It was true, she was tormented by her lovers, who played with her affections. She was always just recovering or just falling. It seemed so poetic, and yet so tiring. I was glad for the safe haven of my life with Richard, and for the day-to-day excitement of the next man, and the next.

THE VIRGIN

It was a fishbowl, the café we worked in. Punters rushed, flinging money across the shiny metal counter. I spilled coffee on them in return, anemic coffee, mostly milk, froth like hairdos used to be, high, air-filled. Crap coffee. They weren't paying us enough.

"They're not paying us enough," he told me, the boy who pulled the coffees, and I agreed.

He was gay. He didn't know it, but he was gay.

"I don't know if I'm gay," he'd say when we dragged ourselves out into the oily inner-city air and filled our lungs with the thick sludge of nicotine and gas fumes. I'd roll my eyes.

"My partner's gay," I told him, which just confused him. The very idea of sex was complex enough for him. Now he had layer upon layer of complications for his imagination to deal with. He puffed away on his cigarette and glanced at me, an accusation.

"I'll never find love," he moaned. "I'm too shy. I'll never go to bed with anybody, ever. I can't even have a conversation with someone in a bar."

I took him to a bar. We had a conversation.

"See?" I told him. "Easier than you knew."

Later, after, I didn't kiss him. I knew him from the fishbowl; he was a friend of mine. He laughed because he had never been naked with anyone before and he was nervous. I laughed because we might have been drinking tea together or baking scones. Richard wasn't laughing. I could feel the slight tremor in his hand as he stroked my friend's solid hip with his fingertips. I had always brought straight boys home for us to play with. Now there was this man, my friend, my virgin gay offering.

"But," nervous, giggling, "see, I don't know if I'm gay or straight or anything."

"Don't be so prescriptive."

I settled my hips, my legs straddling his wide lap. He was all de Lempicka edges, solid curves. I almost kissed him out of habit. It's easy to kiss someone when you are on their lap and their penis has slipped inside you. It's comforting. But tomorrow we would go out for a smoke and there would be a kiss hovering between us and it would make for awkward conversation. Instead I set up a rhythm, kneeling up, settling down and soon Richard was behind me and inside me, too, and leaning over and around and the two of them nuzzling at my breast, using my nipple as an excuse to brush their lips together, their tongues shy as anemones, venturing out to lick and suck and pretending that the kiss they eventually came to was some kind of accident.

At some point I became superfluous. I rolled aside and my body was no longer the point at which they collided. I watched their twin condoms, both moist with the scent of me, tapping against each other, little wet kisses of their own. I lay back and watched and felt fond. Nice men, both of them, and I was glad that now, briefly, through the thin veil of my skin, they had found each other. There was still wine, and I sipped at it, leaning back against the cold sweat of the concrete wall.

When Richard moved too fast, forcing my friend back against the pillow, making clumsy excited lunges too quick, too soon, I leaned toward them, placed my hands on both their chests and felt their wildly beating hearts slow a fraction. Mistress of ceremonies. Nothing more. But I took care. Care with the lubrication. Care with the contraception. Care with the postcoital hugging and the herbal tea by the bed, with three mismatched teacups painted with flowers.

Careful, too, not to wake Richard when my friend crept away before dawn. Careful not to say a word at smoko. Lighting his cigarette from the tip of my own. Smiling, winking, a little nudge with my hip to make him smile, my transient friend who never again wondered about his gender preference and who never again found himself naked in my bed.

I NEED TO TALK ABOUT
FRANK'S PENIS

We never mentioned the size of Frank's penis. It was there before us, thicker than it was long, a little stump of a thing, so wide that the condom barely stretched to fit around it. I'd never seen a penis like it. He took off his jeans and there it was and there was nothing to be said about it, this little mushrooming of flesh.

We paused, Richard and I. The sight of it broke our rhythm. We were used to the routine with each new lover. I would be there first, the comfort of the familiar female flesh pressing and touching and licking my way across the stranger's body. Richard would follow the path that I had cleared for him. Richard was always more gentle than I, easing our lover into the idea of the two of us together, one after the other, my rough urgency, Richard's gentle patience.

Now with the sight of this penis, I faltered. It was uncomfortably wide. It was as thick and oversized as something that Robert Crumb might draw in his pornographic comics, but hacked off short like someone had taken the scissors to the thing, some furious girlfriend, jealous wife, keeping the better part of it as a trophy.

We didn't mention his penis. Richard found the lubrication, gentled the man, what was his name? Yes. Frank. Eased Frank up behind me. The thing felt like a fist, pummeling, butting up against the resistance of flesh. Without the lube it would have been impossible, and yet, with each breach of the battlements, there was a quick retreat, little fist, pounding away like that. I was too startled to find any kind of pleasure.

When it was done, Richard eased him away from me and I watched him change the condom, slipping the thing on with his teeth like a whore. He had learned that trick from me and he had mastered it. I watched the stretch of his mouth. No chance of a gag reflex this time. I wondered how he could do it with a penis like that. It must be like suckling an amputated limb.

Afterward, when Frank left, grinning, touching, kissing too eagerly at the door, we didn't mention his penis. I sat with my cup of tea cooling in my lap and wondered if he even knew how startling it was. How did men get a sense of proportion anyway? It was easy for me, easy for Richard, too, to measure one against the next in the cup of our palms. I had no preference, as long as the thing was not big enough to tear me. Smaller gave us more options. More room for play.

Frank's penis wasn't exactly small though. Huge, from one perspective, and then barely there from a different angle. I wanted to talk to Richard about it but it is difficult to discuss the size of a man's penis.

"He has a good sense of humor."

Richard nodded, sipping, curling back into the lounge chair. His own penis had subsided now and lay like a fat and sated worm in his lap.

"Nice cologne. Expensive. Did you smell it?"

"Yes," I lied. "Very nice."

"And a particularly nice shirt. Good taste. Frank has good taste."

It was impossible to mention his penis. Richard talked about Frank's shoes and his underpants and the way he danced and somehow, reducing the man to the size of his penis seemed petty to me.

"Yes," I said. "He was a good dancer."

"I'd like to see him again." Richard smoothed the little piece of paper out on his knee. There was a telephone number scrawled across it. His number. The man with the little fist of a penis, what was his name? Frank. Frank's little stub of a penis. Already I couldn't remember the way he danced or his cologne or his underwear. All of it obliterated by the blunt fact of his penis, fisting me.

"I think we should invite him over for dinner."

I nodded, calm. Didn't you see the size of his penis? I screamed silently, and, Penis, what about his penis!

We didn't talk about it. We finished our tea and lay politely side by side on the king-size futon with enough distance between his back and mine so that we would never need to mention Frank's penis.

MEETING BRIAN

Richard wouldn't like him. I didn't like him. He was older than us, late forties perhaps, but he dressed like we did. Op-shop clothes, badly fitting, barely ironed. He ordered cappuccinos and the froth crept up onto his upper lip and stayed there. He smiled with his whole face but somehow his eyes were untouched by it. I kept my distance and he kept coming back each afternoon, ordering cappuccinos, glancing over his frothy moustache, grinning at me.

"He wants to sleep with you," Laura whispered under the shriek of the coffee grinder.

"Richard would hate him."

And I was only vaguely interested. I had never slept with a much older man, but I assumed that Brian would be well practiced at his age.

He could perhaps teach me a few things. I was not ready to completely discount the possibility.

He asked me to sit down with him and I couldn't find a reason to refuse. I had finished my shift. I was almost ready to walk across the bridge and home to West End. It had been days since our last conquest and we had begun to tire of our coupledom. The same conversations, the same easy meals. We had started to snipe at each other out of boredom.

He sat and stared and waited; I was expected to say something to him. He was like a particularly attentive puppy hoping for a treat. I was supposed to ask about him, and I did. His name was Brian and he sold coffee to offices for their filter machines and he worked out of his car and he lived out of his car. He did not have a house to go to. I felt the thaw begin. There was something poignant and vulnerable about the man. He was gormless. People didn't really like him. I didn't really like him, but somehow that made me like him. He seemed nice enough in his own way. He seemed to like everybody. He ordered me another coffee and insisted that he should pay.

"I live with a gay man and we share partners," I heard myself saying. "You can sleep on our couch."

Laura raised an eyebrow as I left with him and I shrugged. This was the way it worked, no conscious decisions, just a floating between things. He led me to his car which smelled of aftershave and hair products and just a hint of sweat. He kept it neat, the blankets in a pile folded onto one seat. Too neat perhaps. He held up his key ring with a single key dangling from it.

"One key," he said. "Simplicity."

I jingled my little stash of keys at him. "Shop, house, garage, gate, briefcase, I don't know what that one is, I think that's the key to the last house I lived in and maybe that's the one to the house before."

He shook his head at me, slipped his one key into the ignition, and started the car.

Richard didn't like him. I lay with Richard in our cold king-size bed and there was space between us. My hand snaked out and held his hip, thin as a teenage girl. Sometimes I imagined I could suffocate him if I chose the top position.

"So you won't have sex with him?"

"No."

We kept our voices low because Brian was asleep on the couch just outside. We weren't used to this kind of whispered conversation. Richard reached out and hooked his fingers into my vagina. He did this for comfort. I didn't expect it to be the beginning of anything but it was possible. I imagined that it would be fun to keep our lovemaking a secret. It would add an extra thrill to the play. I shuffled closer and cradled the flaccid curl of his penis in my palm.

"This is the first time you've said no, Richard."

"Well he's old. I don't like that he's old. Old enough to be my father. I couldn't possibly fuck an old man."

"Not so old. You'll be that old one day."

"Okay, I'll fuck him when I'm fifty."

"He'll be dead when you're fifty."

"Do you want to fuck him?"

I thought about that for a while. The possibility. Not something I was longing for, but not so bad. He was older, but he wasn't an old man yet. He smelled all right.

"I want to fuck you," I said.

He could have. I felt his penis begin to stiffen in my fist, but he didn't. He turned away and shuffled his tiny hips so that they were cradled in my generous lap.

"I just want to sleep," he told me.

We lay like that as the night set in and I heard the creaking of the couch as Brian shifted one way or another. I was awake. Wide awake. I wished we had made love, Richard and I. I felt like this might have been some trouble between us and I needed some assurance, flesh to flesh, a quick kiss and make up.

PILLION 3

Brisbane 2008

Of course we will not jump in the spa bath together. This will not happen. I am not even sure that I like him very much. We sit and we drink wine and we talk and the rain gets heavier and heavier.

"I think I'll ride home after all."

Which is ridiculous given the weather and I see Paul cast around frantically for an escape. There are women with cars. He quickly negotiates an alternative to the motorcycle and I am glad, because it will be suicide to ride in this weather, no visibility, dodgy tires, no wet weather gear. I am also disappointed because somewhere on our trip back it would become impossible and we would be stranded at the side of the highway and we would have to huddle together for warmth.

I gather my still-sodden jacket and helmet. I glance at the room with the spa, which is right there near the entrance to the house. I wave goodbye. I do not hug Paul although I feel perhaps we should shake hands. I move out toward the bike and clip the forlorn spare helmet onto the side. The lining will be soaked by the time I have found my way home.

The rattle of tires skidding on wet gravel. I can't see a thing. My right index finger becomes a windscreen wiper for my visor. Even this just makes the world a blur of light and shade. I flip open the visor and the rain pierces my eyeballs. I will look into them and see the bruising on them, on the skin around them, when I am safely home.

Safely home after an hour and a half of breathless terror. It was never worth the risk. I should have stayed the night.

But then there was that spa bath. I dream it. It becomes a recurring theme for the next few nights. We come to it fully clothed, Paul and I, drinking, laughing, acting like children in the early hours of the morning.

Still. I barely know him and I barely like him. Perhaps I don't like him at all. I see Paul's little green light pop up on the Internet and I could talk to him. I could ask him how his lift home was. Instead I close my computer and reach for my sodden book and ease the pulp of pages apart. Tonight I will not chat with him. Tonight I will read, or I will write. Anything but chat.

I close my eyes and all I can see is a spa bath, a glass of wine, and bubbles.

CRACKS

Brisbane 1989

Richard bought a car at an auction although neither of us could drive.

He was always buying things. He had a way of making money disappear. I was barely capable of keeping track of the rent but he was worse than I was.

"Let's eat out," he'd say, meaning a fine restaurant and perhaps a new shirt to wear to it, and the most expensive meal on the menu. He bought me gifts that I didn't want. Kitschy little things, oil burners and homoerotic prints and subscriptions to expensive gay porn magazines. I felt myself digging my heels in, feeling responsible. I was not his mother and yet he made me like a mother to him, always setting boundaries, the voice of reason.

"It's always up to me to find our partners," I complained to Laura one day after a shift. "I never see him put any effort in. If it were up to him it would be just him and me."

Just him and me. I could see the humor in it. Just him and me should not be so bad really, but when I thought about this possibility, all the life seemed to escape out of the relationship.

"You love him, don't you?"

I couldn't be sure I really loved him at all. I loved what I did with him. I loved the potential of our relationship. We had fun. It was exciting, but I had lost my drive to go out every night in search of fresh blood, and our evenings alone together left me irritable.

Brian moved off the couch and into the spare room. We didn't charge him rent but he brought us food and vegetables and I began to enjoy the distraction of him being around. He did the washing and helped with meals. Sometimes when I snapped at Richard in frustration, Brian would be there to pull me aside.

"Let's go for a drive," he said one particularly restless Sunday afternoon.

My final assignments were due and I should have been working, but I was raging about one thing or another and I knew that the afternoon would start to plummet if I didn't leave the house. It had been days since we'd had anyone. I felt cooped up, I had started to pace in the evenings.

"You look like you need your fix."

Brian parked at the edge of the Botanical Gardens. We would

walk, he told me. We would smell the herb garden and maybe steal some cuttings to plant in our own.

"What fix would that be?"

"Someone to distract you from the problems with your own relationship? Sex. Sex with some complete stranger to make you guys feel like you are not all alone with each other."

He seemed like a wise man then, someone twice my age and just as perceptive. He had been in our home for a handful of days and he had put his finger right on the problem, our problem, that we didn't love each other enough.

I felt his hand on my knee and it was a comforting weight.

"I'm tired," I told him. "University is almost over. I don't know what I'm going to do next."

When his finger inched inside the elastic of my panties it was unexpected. I hadn't felt any kind of sexual energy between us. I didn't find him attractive and I had decided that he didn't find me attractive either, but here was his finger inside me, teasing me, changing my mind about my own attraction to him so easily.

"You want to sleep with us?" I asked him, shifting my hips closer to the driver's side of the car and spreading my knees for him. He slipped a second finger inside and slid it back and forth.

"No," he said. "But I wouldn't mind sleeping with you alone."

This was against the rules, our rules, the rules that I had set for both of us. The rules that Richard had agreed to.

When Brian removed his finger he held it to his nose and then he sniffed at it and he wanted me. This made me want him back.

"Have sex with me," he said then and I could hear the desire in his voice.

"I won't break our rules," I told him. "I won't sleep with someone without telling Richard first."

"Are you going to tell Richard?"

"I think this thing with Richard might be over."

"You won't regret it."

"Maybe," I said. "We'll see."

MOVING HOUSE

My assignments were due all at once and I was moving house. This is how university ended for me. This is how Richard ended for me. There was no struggle, but he cried and I felt responsible. I was fond of him. We had shared so much and with such good humor. We packed our things and I hid myself away in the library at night. I needed more time for my work. I was doing too many things badly, and I watched my relationship crumble and I thought perhaps I should have put more effort in.

"We've had fun, haven't we?" And of course we had. So much fun.

There was a twinge of terror in me that this would be the end of sex. We had shared a new partner every week at least and the game had lasted a year. I could have counted them out, averaged them, but I was never good at counting and it wasn't about the numbers, it was about the game, the variety, the smorgasbord. Richard was the safe place from which to begin our adventure. Now it was time to climb back down to the world where everything might be more ordinary. I thought perhaps that I was making a mistake. Brian lurked in the other room, watching us pack, whispering to me that I was making the only choice I could under the circumstances.

Richard left first and I thought this would be a good thing, barely remembering the cleaning and the scrubbing that would have to happen in his absence. Without Richard there was more time for my assignments, and then there was Brian.

He was much older than me and I had a strange kind of respect for the man. He was full of secrets and a manner that seemed to come from another time. He ate his food with his arms hunched around his plate, and once when I picked a piece of tomato off his plate, knowing that he didn't really like tomatoes anyway, he turned and roared like a bear defending her cubs. I was floored by it.

"It's just the army," he explained. "My time in Vietnam."

Vietnam seemed like such a mythical thing to me, the subject of movies and novels, a world of protest and world-changing and politics that I barely understood. Was he even old enough to have gone to Vietnam? When I questioned him about it he snapped shut like a clam and no amount of poking or shaking could rouse him.

We had sex and he told me that I was doing it the wrong way. Not my technique, which he said he enjoyed, but my habit of watching my partner's actions, memorizing it all, then finding a greater pleasure when I was alone. He said that I should make noises. That this would free me from my inhibitions. He took away my vibrator saying that I should come to an orgasm simply by being in the moment. None of this made sense to my body and I found that I became self-conscious with it. The noises sounded fake and distracted me. Orgasms proved elusive. I almost had them and then they would slip away and leave me longing for my vibrator.

I was not used to this kind of exclusiveness, this one on one, and I began to misinterpret it. I made the mistake of calling him "my boyfriend" and he pounced on me.

"You are not a girlfriend kind of person," he told me, another in a long line. "If I were to have a girlfriend she would be an earth mother kind of girl. You are too hard edged, too manly."

I felt the hackles rising on my neck. We fought. There was nothing wrong with me, I said. I was honest and dependable and smart.

"I want someone feminine, someone with secrets. You have no secrets. You are empty and there is nothing about you that I have yet to learn."

We fought in the car on the freeway and his temper was formidable. I watched him close his eyes and lean forward on the accelerator.

I laughed at him then and every time he performed this trick for me, which was often.

"Go on," I said. "Kill us. Do you think I care if you kill us?"

I didn't care. I looked ahead past my university degree and there was just the café where I worked and more sex, but not enough, never enough sex and no bright and shining future to walk into. He stepped on the accelerator and closed his eyes and I said, "Bring it on. Kill us both now. Do it." And he swore and hissed and eased back to a safer speed.

"You'd better find a house to move to," he said in the last week at Ryan Street.

"What about you?"

He held up his key, his single key.

"You won't move in with me somewhere?" and he laughed as if I had offered to chop off his head for him.

"I would rather move in with your friends," he told me, listing the women I knew one by one and telling me why each one would be a better choice than me.

He took his one key and he left me on my knees scrubbing the oven.

"Need anything from the shop?"

I looked up and wiped my forehead. He was leaving. Somehow I knew he was leaving and it would be just me and the oil-encrusted oven and the removalists in a few days and nowhere in particular to go.

"A cleaning lady," I told him and he laughed.

"You look great in rubber gloves you know."

And then he left.

He's gone, I thought. I struggled out of the rubber gloves and I walked to the door of his room and the few possessions that he owned were gone. I sat on his bed in the sour smell of his sheets and I rode a surge of anger, and then loneliness and then loss. When it was over I dragged myself to my feet and settled down with my head in the oven. The irony was not lost on me. I laughed, coughed from the lungful of chemical reek, and settled back to the task at hand.

NOT TALKING ABOUT
THE SPA BATH

Brisbane 2008

Paul is there.

It is late and I am sleepless and he is there on my computer screen, a little box with his word flashing there as if he has spoken. Cleared his throat, and said,

Hi.

And I imagine it is said with a kind of bounce. Just one word but there is a kind of energy about it that makes me think he might be grinning. I had decided not to speak with him.

I have decided not to speak with you.

Why?

Because we fought.

Did we?

There is no voice to the line of text that appears on the screen but I imagine his innocent upward inflection. He seems so keen and quick and gormless. I remind him that he likes the only three girls who dislike me.

Oh, I like everyone, he says, and I think it's probably true.

Did you see the spa bath? I ask him. If I had stayed the night I might have had a spa bath.

Yeah, he says, me, too.

A silence can't be awkward on the Internet. A silence is an indication that one person or another is busy looking up a website, or answering an email or ducking off to the kitchen for another glass of wine.

Still, I imagined the minutes that followed this, empty of conversation, as a kind of embarrassed silence. Certainly I filled them with the idea that the two of us might have stripped down to our underwear and eased ourselves into the spa. Twin glasses perched on the sudsy lip of the bath, talking about the difference between the short form and the novel, the way a story circles around a single thought, the multiple thoughts and voices of a longer work.

I am playing the scene out in my head when Paul types, I am on the phone, and I realize that he would never want to share a spa bath with me, clothed or otherwise. He is fifteen years younger than I am. He sees me as an elder, perhaps. Someone interesting to talk to with nothing even remotely sexual about it.

It is time perhaps to admit that I have developed a little crush on him, despite the way he annoys me in real life. I know too well that if I keep this thing a secret it will grow in size and intensity until it becomes unbearable. I must stop falling in love with my friends.

Paul is on the phone. This is why there is a gaping hole in our conversation, but suddenly the silence is deafening.

Okay, then I should go.

Really?

Yes. Maybe we'll meet in real life again some time.

Next week.

Really?

Thursday evening?

Okay.

Okay.

And then I close my computer and he is gone.

SPRING HILL

Brisbane 1990

Two of the beautiful women at work had a room coming free. Jessica was the cold, quiet one and there was something about her I distrusted. Her silence seemed like a provocation, a passive flirtation. She giggled too easily at jokes that weren't funny and she always seemed to have a group of young men hovering around her, waiting to alight.

Mary seemed far more sophisticated than I was. She worked as a part-time model when she wasn't pulling coffees, and when I saw her in a glossy magazine I thought she was more startling than the other girls. She was lovely and quietly spoken and hopeless in her choice of lovers, always falling for someone who would treat her badly. The Nina Simone songs that my friend Laura played seemed to speak of Jessica's life, which was so beautiful and tragic. She was committed to a cultish self-help group called the Living Game and I couldn't help but imagine that this was a little like her bad relationships: a charismatic leader like her charismatic boyfriends who would one day leave her broken and weeping.

The day I moved into their Spring Hill house they were playing the Cocteau Twins on vinyl. They had a CD player and a tape deck and a record player so old it would play 78s. I was tired and sweating from lugging boxes alongside the delivery men, and they had iced fruit punch. They turned the music up too loud and we danced. Jessica moved too close to me and pressed herself up against me and it was not like the joyful prancing that I shared with Laura. It was something about the smell of her and her slow, languid movements, and her cool stare. She caught my eye and then, having my full attention, looked slyly away. I really didn't trust her, and I danced away from her and excused myself to shower. But I was still caught in her sly gaze.

I removed the shower hose and pressed it against myself until I came with the sweet dewberry scent of her bath products in my nostrils.

I hadn't shared a house with women since I lived at Dragonhall. These girls were not the practical kind of women I was used to. They shopped for clothes and staged impromptu fashion parades, sometimes in expensive underwear and little else.

I watched, entranced. They were beautiful and I lived in a constant state of excitement. I sniffed their face creams and their powders and their makeup, I had never worn makeup and they sat me down in a comfortable chair and made me lean back while they painted my eyes. When I looked in the mirror I was unrecognizable.

Sometimes we dressed for dinner. We put on our op-shop gowns and stockings and high heels. We spent hours on our hair and nails and cooked a three-course fantasy. I had never eaten desserts as part of a daily routine; the girls loved dessert. They loved chocolate. They bought bright bunches of flowers and filled the house with scent. There was always some woman crooning on the record player. There was always dancing.

On the nights when they went to their Living Game seminars they tried to talk me into accompanying them.

"You are such an enlightened soul," they pleaded. "I'm sure you will love it."

Of course I wouldn't. "I have no soul," I said. "I don't believe in a soul."

They returned from the seminars with stories of great feats of daring, fears they had overcome. They had snapped an arrow by running into it. They had walked over hot coals. They wrote affirmations and stuck them up on the toilet door: I am strong; I am beautiful; I am the goddess; I am a divine representation of the universe.

I copied my favorite lines from books I had been reading. Every portrait that is painted with feeling is a portrait of the artist, not of the sitter—Oscar Wilde. Each generation imagines itself to be more intelligent than the one that went before it, and wiser than the one that comes after it—George Orwell. I stuck them up amongst their platitudes and it was clear that I would not be attending the Living Game.

"You should come to the sex seminar," they told me. "You would love it."

Jessica described a three-day retreat spent almost completely naked where you divulged your worst sexual fears and then worked to overcome them—where you opened yourself up to all the universe had to offer. It sounded more like a compulsory group orgy where no one was allowed to refuse physical contact with any other participant.

When Jessica was gone I thought about her. I crept into her room and lay down on her pillow and inhaled the scent of her hair. I moved down the mattress picking out the individual odors, I curled about the place where it smelled of her sex and rubbed myself till I came. I washed myself with her soap and her shampoo. I filled in my lips with her pearly color but it was too pale for my skin tone. We were mismatched, it seemed: still I missed her. I cooked a welcome-home meal for both of them, peering through the curtains looking for the flash of her blond hair.

She had a boyfriend of sorts. He was a part of the Living Game and although he adored her, he was practicing non-monogamy for the good of his soul. When he visited I saw him follow her compulsively with the sticky trail of his gaze. He is in love, I thought, without realizing that I had developed the same habit of turning my head toward her.

One night she came to find me. I was curled up with the fireplace blazing. My room was at the bottom of the terrace house. The bricks were left exposed which gave the space a dark and homey feel. There was a beam of wood running across the middle of each wall and I had filled this with images I had drawn. I had my sketch pad in my lap and my music playing and she was there in the doorway. I was imagining her into the fallen angel on my sketch pad and then she was there.

She came into my room and pulled back the bedclothes to crawl inside. She smelled of sex. Her boyfriend had been visiting and it was there behind the floral scent of perfume and hair products. She nestled into my shoulder and I held myself stiff and tight beside her. There was yellow ochre on my fingers, thick slivers of black oil pastel under my nails. My room was untidy, with piles of books toppling in every corner, pages thick with paint drying on the sisal carpet. She held her arm up against mine and measured the difference between them.

It was easy. She was cream and silk, I was oil and hessian. She was everything that I was not, compliant, soft, scented, warm. She was the type of girl that men would want as their girlfriend, and I was not the girlfriend kind.

"You okay?" I asked her and she nestled in closer.

She seemed small and vulnerable. I wondered if this was what men wanted in a woman, this sense of defenselessness. It would make you feel useful, a protective force for someone who truly needs you. I slipped my arm around her. I knew that this was her aim, the spell that she was casting on me. I was not blind to it. I knew that it was just a trick she had learned from being so beautiful.

I began to feel sorry for her, born with such a body and such a face. She would never need to develop her humor or her intelligence. She would be required to sit around looking decorative. Poor Jessica. Poor sweet Jessica and all her lost potential.

"What is it like to sleep with two men at once?"

This was the most complete sentence I had ever heard her utter. She was full of giggles and vague, trailing replies. I had made her use a whole sentence. I felt special, and even as I felt it I knew I was being manipulated into feeling special.

"It's fun. That was probably the most fun I have ever had. You know, I think maybe it was a mistake to abandon it so quickly. I don't miss Richard, but I miss what we did together. Maybe I'll never have that kind of fun again."

"I think you should." A pause. "Should with me."

Should with me.

It was not exactly a complete sentence but it was enough to make me want to roll onto her right then, heart pounding, and slip my fingers into her cunt. It was all I could do to keep the little distance there was. I was drunk with the idea of sex with her.

"Me and Laura," she said and I felt the pause in my chest, the insecurities creeping back.

"Three girls?"

"Three girls and a boy."

"Which boy?"

"Someone. Someone we all approve of."

There were warning bells of course, but when she rolled to the edge of my bed and slipped off it, there was still that smell of her sex, which was half almond paste, half golden syrup and completely intoxicating.

"Does Laura know about this?"

She nodded and giggled. They had spoken about it in my absence. I tried to imagine the conversation. I tried to imagine how they had come to the idea. Perhaps it was at the Living Game, the sex seminar. I could imagine Laura talking about my adventures with my various boys. She had always been interested. Perhaps she had brought it up in a group situation, all of them sitting around and disclosing the intimate details about their sex lives. My sex life. I didn't mind, I had nothing to hide. But I wondered how it would work, this choosing a boy by committee. In the other time, with Richard, it was all my choice and he rarely vetoed any of them, he was just happy to be supplied with new lovers night after night.

"So," she hovered in my doorway. The light loved her. She caught it beautifully, her hair, her skin, her subtle curves. I watched the way the last of the sunlight found its way through my window and could not keep its hands off her body.

I nodded. "Sure. I'm in if you are."

She grinned and was gone, but I had the scent of her sex captured under my bedcovers. I had the fading heat of her. One day soon, if we could manage the correct combination of components, I would have my fingers inside her. I sighed and pulled the blankets up over my head and breathed in deeply.

THREE GIRLS AND AN APOLOGY

I had agreed to it because I wanted to sleep with them. Both of them, but mostly with her, Jessica. They were both beautiful, though Jessica was blond and Laura a sandy brown and my hair was a darker chestnut color. Something for everyone I suppose. I looked at the two of them, breasts so pillowy that it was all I could do to stop myself touching them, easing those breasts out of their twin plunging necklines into my palms. I wanted Jessica with a kind of dull ache deep in the guts of me, and Laura would take some of the edge off it. She would keep it light, a game.

"But not until we find a man who will sleep with the three of us together. Someone we all three agree on. It has to be someone we agree on."

We listed names one after the other. Men we all wanted (one

name). Men we could all tolerate (two names). Men one or the other of the girls would absolutely refuse to sleep with (a whole list of names stretching out over four blank pages). I didn't veto anyone. I just wanted to sleep with the two of them together. The identity of the man seemed like a detail.

One of the tolerable two found himself at our kitchen table with Jessica and me. We told him the plan and I did the talking, as always. She watched him carefully and I watched her, my heart an erratic mix of beats in my chest. I would sleep with her. Soon I would sleep with her.

The boy seemed amenable to the idea, and he, like myself, wanted to ease Jessica's plunging neckline down just a little. I watched as he reached across the table, fumbling with the sheer fabric and I wished I had just got right down to it without waiting to be invited. His head fit snugly between the rise and fall of them. I saw peach fuzz, a flash of nipple-pink. She giggled. She seemed to enjoy the attention for a moment, then slipped away from the kneading of his fingers and settled herself back inside her dress. I felt a shot of saliva wet the inside of my mouth. I could almost feel the hard little nub of pink nipple butting against the back of my throat. It took me a moment to realize I had stopped breathing.

She told him to wait. We would wait for Laura to come around after work.

The boy leaned back in his chair and locked eyes with me and lifted an eyebrow. I knew what he meant and he knew that I knew and I had found an unexpected ally in all of this. I could already see us down at the pub with a postcoital beer, discussing the ins and outs of the thing, comparing notes as if we had just sat through a game of football.

When we were finally in bed, he gave me a wink as if to say, "How good is this?" It was indeed fine. The girls were like unwrapped presents, pink and drenched in perfume and with hair that spilled out over each other's chests. Every part of them was fragranced. Each strand of hair dripping sweetness, the smooth shaved skin under their arms, the underside of the necks, both blooming with scent.

I would be a contrast to them. I would underline their femininity with my musky skin. My nipples olive, my flesh a dirty tan, my hair too rough and wiry to run fingers through. I kissed them each in turn, soft kisses scented with Cointreau, orange blossom tongues, the hard line of their teeth, and suddenly it was his mouth against mine. The boy that we could all tolerate. A battle of lips and cheeks and the roughness of his re-emerging stubble. He measured the generous bulk of my breasts in his palms and I wondered suddenly if he had chosen my mouth because I was a relief amongst this paradise of girl-flesh. He moved behind me and he was inside me in a second. I suppose I was the easiest beginning for him. I was his place of entry and he took it. No preamble, no negotiation, just a sliding inside, a reaching over my shoulder. In this position he would not be in my way, and I returned to the promise of breasts, with an animal urge to suckle, an overpowering need to bite down on the pillowy swell. I felt his finger pinch the flesh that I was licking, I felt a thumb in my mouth. He was reading my actions like Braille, touching the hard nipple, the soft wetness of my tongue. He was there at the point of our connection. He entered me and I entered her, just a finger at first but I was surprised by the moisture, a deluge. She was so wet and pink and open to me and I wanted to be inside her. I arched my back and bent my head down and she filled up my senses. I pressed my fingers together as if I were about to dive and some of them slipped inside her as I traced the little protrusion of her clitoris. The boy behind me pushed with a rhythm that was not mine and I shoved back at him, as if trying to kick aside the annoyance of a puppy, bouncing and spilling things. I had completely lost track of Laura but she was there somewhere, doing something. It didn't matter to me. I was buried in Jessica.

And then . . .

My face felt a cold rush of air and the girl was gone. She had slipped out from under me. I felt the void rushing toward me, like when you are small and you lie on your back on the grass and look up at the night sky contemplating the size of the universe. The disappointment of her loss was universal. I couldn't be sure what had occurred but they were gone, both of them, the girls. There was just me and him and he didn't even pause in his pounding. The hot space where her body had been touching mine turned icy in a second. I kneeled in the bed and watched them leave the room as the boy continued to grunt and sweat and paw at me.

I strained to listen to the conversation playing out in the kitchen. I wouldn't be able to come. I knew that this thudding of bodies had nothing to do with my pleasure. I wanted to be in the kitchen with the girl talk, but there was this boy and the disappointment of a plan abandoned and I settled back into the comfort of simple, uncomplicated girl-on-boy coupling.

I turned over and brought my feet up onto his chest and felt the place where his penis connected with my flesh, pressed the palm of my hand hard onto my clitoris. My hand smelled of her. My hand was wet with her. I covered my face with one hand and there was her pink sex open to me and my tongue snaking out onto my fingers to taste her and I came so violently that he was forced to dig his fingers into my hips to hold his place.

He spasmed and he was coming and in the hazy place after an orgasm I fumbled vaguely for a name to call him by. He opened his mouth and would have spoken, but I held a finger to my lips.

We rolled apart and listened. It felt as if we were having an affair and the wives were in the next room drinking tea and debriefing (endlessly debriefing) what we had begun together but were finishing without them. We dressed quietly and when we stood in the door of the kitchen we could tell there had been tears and talking, but they glared at us, red eyes dry, mouths stitched shut. They pulled their satiny robes around their soft pink bodies. I wondered why I didn't have a satiny robe. I sat beside the tolerable boy and listened as they explained the impossibility of it all to us. We nodded and made calming sounds, little grunts and sighs that made us seem understanding and sympathetic. They started from the beginning and explained it all again and again but none of it made any sense.

We had done something wrong. Something had happened to contravene some rule or another. I tried to think back to the moment when it all fell apart, but all I could see was her sex, wet and open and the scent of fruit and flowers and something more true and earthy hidden beneath it.

"It's not a particular thing," Laura told me. "It's just the energy of it."

I caught Jessica's eyes, expecting a knowing acknowledgment of what had passed between us, but there was just fire and steel and silence.

"But what exactly went wrong?" I was confused. "What actually happened?"

They looked toward each other, exasperated, and shook their heads to show that I would never understand even though it was perfectly obvious.

Eventually I yawned. "I should walk him to his car." I rested a sympathetic hand on both of their shoulders. They said nothing.

I would never understand the complicated pattern of quickly shifting emotional threads that girls spin quick as spiderweb. I would never be a real girl. Not like these girls.

"I feel like a beer," I told him when the door was safely shut behind us, "and a cigarette."

He nodded. "The pub's just down the road."

We sat at the pub and I lit his cigarette from the end of mine and we drank beer.

"Well, that was something," he said, and I grinned.

We sat and drank beer and said nothing until I remembered something I'd read in the paper about experiments with rats and mazes, and he had read it, too. We talked about that until our glasses were empty. We hugged awkwardly, like blokes hug, stiff bodies bouncing off each other, and then he got in his car and drove home. I tried, but I couldn't remember his name.

"I'll see you later then," I told him.

"Yeah, matey. See you then," he said.

THE GIRL I ONCE LOVED

Something had subtly changed. We still cooked elaborate dinners. We still dressed in evening gowns and set the table with candles. We still went to work at the café and shared our shifts, one of them or another crowded beside me in a cramped space, but it was different now. I watched her more closely. She knew she was being watched and played a fascinating game.

She invited me to bathe with her. I lowered myself into the scented bubbles with shaking hands but she kept her knees clamped tight against her chest and I only caught glimpses of her. She barely spoke a word to me the whole time we were soaking.

We were asked to be in a music video and the director told me to reach over to her, to fondle her breasts and then to kiss her. I couldn't seem to pull away when the director yelled cut.

Sometimes when we were walking in the street, a boy would pass us on the other footpath and she would reach for my hand, or nuzzle into my shoulder or even kiss me with her lips parted, locking her fingers into the crazy wire of my hair until the boy was out of sight and she could walk on without comment.

I watched her when she wandered down the hill to the city, the sunlight outlining her legs under her white skirt. I watched her sit in front of the television with her knees lolling wide and a little damp line at the center of her pristine white panties. I admired her, I was envious of her, I wanted to be her. And I wanted to fuck her.

One day she came to me. There was sunlight on my bed. It touched my naked legs and I noticed that it didn't reach to where she was stretched out in the dark. Strange that I was all lit up and she was not. On any ordinary day her beauty cast a shadow that obliterated me. We were side by side and we hadn't really touched since that night.

My skin was heated in a sun pattern. I settled my knee against hers. She didn't shift away. My hand was close to her buttons and I touched one with my finger. I struggled it through the tight enclosure of the buttonhole. When it was open I eased my finger into the space, feathered it back and forth. Maybe she felt the gentle rustle of it so close to the swell of her breast.

She didn't move. She didn't shift away when I eased my fingers upward to where another button held the delicate fabric closed across the generous proportions of her breasts. I eased her shirt away and her bra was revealed, thick and delicate as an orchid, her flesh rising above the albino petals.

I unbuttoned my own shirt and gazed down at the inconsistencies of our flesh. Her pale and delicately scented breasts. My generous dark oiled flesh. I wondered if I would ever tire of comparing myself to her.

I eased the cups of my bra down and there were my brown nipples, enlarged areolas, the tight nubs clenched at their peaks. I wished I had thought to pluck away the scattering of dark hairs before revealing myself to her.

She still hadn't moved. I looked to her face, the heavy-lidded eyes gazing down toward those now-erect stray hairs. She hadn't asked me to stop but she hadn't invited my attentions either.

I wanted to show her what to do. I wanted to lead by example. I clutched one of my breasts in my fist and raised it out of the loose droop of my bra cup. I bent my head toward it and I licked the nipple so she could see the flesh grow taut. The nipple ached out toward the touch of tongue like an accusing finger. I took it all into my mouth. I suckled, a show for her, a demonstration. She could lean down and lick it, too, alongside my own mouth. She could replace my attentions with her own. I lifted both of my breasts toward her mouth, so close that her breathing disturbed the fine pale hairs that lined the swell of them. If she were to yawn she would swallow a nipple, but her mouth remained firmly closed. She sighed and settled closer to me. I felt her hips brush mine. My knee was caressed by the fine swell of her calf. She raised her legs.

My hands released my breasts back into their holdings. My fingers traveled the swell of my stomach and touched the elastic of my panties. Her crotch was somewhere down there. I stretched my index finger out and there was the tight press of white cotton, slightly damp but perfectly laundered.

She nestled closer, pushed her crotch against my fingers, closed her eyes and settled where she was within reach of my shivery finger. It was all I could do not to tear away the pretty white cotton, but I restrained myself. I eased my finger under the elastic. She was wet; I felt the same pleasure at this discovery as I had in our brief tussle with the chosen boy.

I wondered whether I dared shuffle down her body and taste the nectar once more. My mouth watered at the thought of it. Her breath was sweet, her skin was sweet, her hair was sweet. I was hoping that her cunt would add a savory edge to a palette that was otherwise all pales and pinks and sugary pastel hues. I moved my fingers into the nest of fine cropped hair. I imagined she trimmed it with scissors. It was so fine and neat, manicured like expensive lawn. I opened her as I had opened her buttons, easing my fingers under the delicate fabric of her skin, fluttering my finger back and forth, making space for the rude invasion of my own flesh. She opened to me, moist and soft and I remembered that she would be seashell pink like the inside of some spidery white mollusc. My tongue itched for mussels, oysters, pipis.

The phone rang. She opened her eyes and stretched and my finger was abandoned to the harsh cold Sunday afternoon air. I shifted back away from the darkness into the spotting of sunlight. She rolled off my king-size bed and I heard her little bird voice from the next room as she answered the phone.

"Hello? No, nothing much. Now's good."

I sniffed my finger, licked it. Sweet. She was sweet. There was no hint of a base note. She was all sugar, all the way through. I shuffled over into the darkness where I smelled her sweat and perfume sweet on the pillow and I curled my damp finger around a single, abandoned, blond hair.

THE STRAIGHT GIRL

There was, of course, her boyfriend. I think he knew that she was flirting with the idea of a lesbian lover. He glared at me jealously across the dinner table whenever we were alone together. There was rarely any conversation between us. Sometimes he would talk about the Living Game and about how only the unenlightened would refuse to take part in it. He kissed her in front of me, open-mouthed.

One afternoon I was reading *Alice in Wonderland* naked in her bed. She was barely clothed. It was summer and our clothes were abandoned by the doorway. I felt her held breath close against the bare skin of my breast. My nipple pulled tighter, inching closer to her slightly parted lips.

I was all wound up. I was reading to her and wondering if we would make love. I needed to make love. This time, I thought, this time we would definitely make love. Then there were his footsteps on the stairs and he was with us.

He had never seen me naked before. She had been naked with us, dripping out from a shower with her hair all dark with scent and water. He had once lifted her onto the kitchen bench and then there was that thing he did with the Lebanese cucumber and I watched, pretending this was the sort of display that all my roommates had treated me to. But he had never seen me even partially unclothed. Now, he was watching from the doorway.

I sensed her turn toward him like a sunflower photosynthesizing. She never turned like that in my direction. The few times that we had made our odd uncompleted kind of love, it had been all me. She might sigh and part her thighs just a little farther, making those little dove sounds at the back of her throat that made me want to bite down on the pillow, tear the sheets, force myself into the perfect peaches and cream of her skin.

So—the sunflower thing, the gentle movement of her body, and there at the apex of her attentions was the boy. Looking at me naked for the first time, my body pressed close to hers, my nipple almost, but not quite, entering her mouth, the pages of *Alice* closing, dropping to the bed beside me.

There was a leveling up, a squaring off. I know I settled my shoulders more firmly on the bed. It was her bed, smaller than my own but with nicer sheets and the scent of roses. I held my ground and he held his, pulling up straighter in his casual lean, filling his chest with air, tensing his shoulders just a little, making him look stronger than he had a moment before. All this alpha stuff that we share with dogs and lions and rats. We might have stayed that way all night if she hadn't snuggled just that little bit closer, latching on to my breast like a suckling child, with that full red pout of her lips that both of us had kissed at one time or another.

He took his clothes off. He settled down beside her, pressing his hips into her. I might have rolled away then and left them, but she was licking my breast and cooing like she did and I knew she wanted me to stay. I wanted to stay. I wanted to leave. I saw him lift her thigh and slide himself into her and I felt an acid burn of jealousy rage through me. I was her show and tell. I was here for her to wave before him and as he started to push himself into her in a rhythm, I hooked glances with him and I could see that same jealous spark burning in him like lust.

He fucked her, and I was aroused by the fucking. I stretched my finger toward her delicate pink cunt and I felt his penis entering her, bare, no condom anywhere to be felt and I remember thinking that I would never let him ride me bareback. I would have to be certain of his fidelity before I opened myself up to that kind of risk. He went to the sex seminars. He played with nonmonogamy. How could she let him be inside her like that, pumping his diseased juices into something so sweet and clean and perfect?

But there was excitement in that kind of risk. I held my fist against my clitoris and rubbed against it. I inserted my fingers into her alongside his penis. I felt his rhythm and timed my own movements to it. When he paused I was close to coming. I kept on at it. I pushed my fingers into myself and rubbed myself and moved my fingers into and out of her. I felt his penis tighten and then pulse. I came. My head kicked back and I squeezed my eyes shut and I wondered if the openness at the moment of orgasm was some animal signal of submission.

When it was over I slid my hand out of her. I couldn't tell if she had come to orgasm. All my attention had been diverted to the palpitations of my own flesh. My fingers were coated in stickiness. It might have been her juices, but perhaps there was some of his semen on them. I wiped them on the sheets. I stood and gathered my clothes and I was at the door when I heard him.

"Sorry," he said to her. "I couldn't stop myself. Someone was moving."

Someone moved now. Down the stairs and into the bathroom and under the scalding heat of the shower I rubbed at the paint stains on my fingers until my nails gleamed and my fingers were prunes.

PICNIC IN A VACANT LOT

I needed to see other people, I thought. I needed to stop obsessively following Jessica from work to home to the supermarket to her bed. I needed a romantic project. I had seen this boy at the restaurant where he worked and I liked the look of him. There was perhaps a moment of flirtation. I wrote the address on a note card. Meet me at—a time and a place. Dress: Formal and had it delivered to him by one of the other staff. High romance.

I thought about him all afternoon as the food was cooking. I took off Jessica's wafty girly music and played old David Bowie as I stirred the sauce. A vegetable lasagne, easy to transport to my picnic spot in the vacant block across the street. It would stay hot wrapped in a tea towel, and if the boy didn't turn up I could take it all back home and offer it to her. We could dine on it for several nights.

It all fit into the one basket: two plates, the cutlery, the food, the wine, and two dozen candles. There was a bit of work in setting the candles in their paper bags. I had to clear away long grass, chip packets, an abandoned shopping trolley. It looked quite pretty when it was done, the picnic blanket in the center of a flickering glow. I had put on an evening gown and heels. Away from Jessica and Mary and our extravagant evenings together, I felt vaguely like I was in drag. The heels sank into the loose earth when I walked and there were insects. I checked my watch and poured myself a glass of wine. He was late. He wouldn't be coming. He was late. I had decided that I should eat my portion anyway and watch the stars. A picnic for one in a vacant lot. I had brought a book and I would read by candlelight.

I was therefore surprised to see him, dressed in a suit. The remarkably comic bow tie should have been a warning for me but I thought he looked quite beautiful. He loomed above me, looking at the world of candlelight that I had created, and had a good laugh. He told me I was completely mad; I poured him a glass of wine.

We picnicked, and then we threw the blanket on top of the dirty plates and kicked dust onto the candles, watching the scraps of paper bag catch fire and drift up toward the sky. The air was alight with hope and there was laughter and holding hands as we headed back across the street.

Jessica met us at the door; I had forgotten my key and Jessica opened the door in her nightgown. She looked like an angel with her perfect body and her halo of brushed blond hair, and I realized, suddenly, that he would want to sleep with her.

I felt him shift and he let my hand slip away. His whole body turned toward her as if she were the fireplace on a cold night. My fingers caught chill and I rubbed them against my thigh to warm them.

Bad to worse.

There is a kind of man who will not use a condom, a generation of boys just a little older than myself who were unmoved by the vision of the grim reaper. We lay naked beside each other. The condom was a little flaccid thing, drooping between my fingers, until, exhausted by negotiation, I let him slip inside me, skin on skin, for just a moment. I lay beneath him with my knees drawn up to my chest and my toes pressing against his nipples and all the joy had gone out of the thing. I pushed him away with my feet. There was the wet sound of our parting. I nestled down to finish the job with my mouth and he told me he liked the idea that I could suck his penis when it was ripe with the taste of my own juices—which, of course, he had not tasted.

"You're a lesbian aren't you? Or bisexual?"

Someone had told him about Jessica. This was all about Jessica.

"So tell me about your roommate," he said.

I pulled away from his long hairless body. A perfect body and a golden mane fanning out on the red satin pillow.

"Are you interested in my roommate?"

"I'm just asking," he said and I watched his perfect penis bounce excitedly at the mention of her.

I eased away.

"She's beautiful," I told him and he agreed. "She's still awake," I said. "You could go talk to her, she'll probably make you a cup of tea."

He was climbing into his suit pants, pushing his erection down under the belt, dragging his collared shirt up and over his head. He stood on my futon, disheveled and beautiful.

"You want a cup of tea?"

I shook my head.

He left the door open as if he was expecting to be back. I closed it, locked it, and lay back on the bed. I thought about the little sparks of burning paper bag floating up into the night sky. There was something underneath me. I scratched up a wormy withered condom. I pulled it back like a slingshot and snapped it up toward the pressed metal ceiling. It arced up, not quite managing to hit the roof, and fell, limp, to the bed beside me.

ON THE TABLE

And then there was the boyfriend's brother.

"Jessica says you will sleep with me if I ask," he said, lounging in my bedroom doorway. All grinning teeth.

Jessica says.

I shrugged and slept with him. A quick, disinterested fuck. When it was over I lay there thinking about her body, wishing he would leave my bed so that I could masturbate in private.

In the morning there she was eating breakfast. A mountain of food, I wondered how she could eat so much and remain so willowy. I watched her flick her long pale hair over her shoulder and I was jealous and desirous all at once. He watched her, too. He was her boyfriend's brother and I could see that this was irrelevant to him.

"I fucked your friend," he said to her. Those teeth bothered me. I couldn't bear them, all spit and sparkle.

She smiled at us as if she approved, and I love-hated her completely.

"Don't you believe me?" he asked her, even though it was clear that she did.

"You told me she'd have sex with me and so she did." I was invisible. It was all about them. I watched her smouldering glance burn through the rich fall of her hair. I wondered when he would leap across the table, pushing aside the chairs and the vase of wilted flowers that I had bought for her and the bowl of cereal and my body, all those items superfluous to the purpose of their conversation. I wondered how long until I saw him kiss her horribly wonderful mouth.

Instead he reached for me and lifted me and put me up on the table for display. He was going to fuck me on the table in front of her. I wasn't certain what my reaction should be. I watched as she paused, placed the spoon back into the bowl. She pushed breakfast to one side and watched us with that half-lidded bored expression she had perfected. She wanted to watch him fucking me on the table. She wanted to watch me being fucked. I wanted her to watch me.

I peeled my shirt off because I wanted her to see my breasts. I bent and suckled on my own breasts because I wanted her mouth there. I was modeling behavior. I hoped that this scene would be repeated without her boyfriend's brother. I wanted her all for myself again.

He was clumsy with my clothing, scratching my thighs with overlong fingernails as he wrestled my panties down. He lifted one of my legs and pointed to my vagina. She looked. I felt her eyes on me, sharper than his finger as he pushed it inside. She was looking at his one finger, two, then three, disappearing inside my body and I wished it was her fingers. I would tolerate her ridiculously manicured nails, I would enjoy the little nips of her talons, tearing at my flesh. I wanted to be this open for her and when he pushed me around and spread my knees for her to see the slightly parted labia, I hoped that she would lean over and look more closely. She didn't.

He turned me back around and plucked one of my condoms from his pocket. He had planned this; he had taken it when he was dressing. He had stood in the shower and thought up the idea of fucking me in front of her.

He fucked me on the table, the brother of her boyfriend, and I was barely even present. It was about him and it was about her, and it was about his brother and whatever had passed between them over the years.

He came before I was ready and it was finished. She pulled her bowl of cereal toward her and continued to eat without a word.

I was suddenly shy. I hadn't had an orgasm. I wanted to be bold enough to turn toward her and show her how my climax might be achieved with a slight fluttering of her fingertip. I wanted to but I didn't. I was suddenly self-conscious as I slid off the table and pulled my pants back on.

Later, in the shower, I barely needed to touch myself. There was the smell of her shampoo on the walls and the slipperiness of her highly scented soap beneath my feet. There was her razor on the soap dish and she had stood naked under the same scald of water. I had to hold the wall with shaking fingertips to stop myself from falling. I heard her little breathy bird-voice in the kitchen, asking some question of the brother of her boyfriend. Have you seen the milk? Do you want another cup of coffee? My clitoris tugged toward the sound of her voice. I held the open cap of her shampoo close to my face and fell a second time, silently sliding to the floor of the shower and placing a hand over the wild race of my heart.

He stayed with us for a week and she orchestrated a nice dance for the three of us. Four of us, because her boyfriend was there with us, too, even though he was physically away at a retreat. She didn't want him to go on the retreat where he would talk about universal consciousness and have sex with other women and extricate himself from her grasp just a little bit. So in her boyfriend's absence there was her boyfriend's brother. I could see the appeal. So many complications and her at the center of it all, with her hands clean and smelling of sweet bath oils. She had a way of making things happen without even touching them.

That day in her bedroom was a surprise. She liked to watch him with me. I let him touch me in front of her because she wanted it. He had crazy eyes and talked with her for hours in phrases from the Living Game. They talked about mantras and affirmations and choosing your disease to teach you universal lessons. I wondered whether a child born with HIV was choosing her own death to learn some kind of lesson. They looked at me blankly, and I knew I would never make sense in their shared game of life. I stopped talking and I started to just watch without listening.

She settled down onto her pillow, lifting the golden mane of hair into her delicate fingers, leaning on her palm and watching. She wanted to watch us. We knew this and he unzipped my skirt and showed my body to her and entered it quickly, all of this for her. She did nothing. She did everything. We heard her little murmurs, the only sign of her pleasure, just a breathy cooing that encouraged us.

I'm not sure who touched her first, but somehow our fingers were slick with her. I remember lifting the damp white cotton of her pants and then I was inside her, he was inside her. Our fingers had fused and they worked in the same rhythm that his hips had found. Her lover's brother, her female lover, and her at the juicy apex of it all.

I remember her orgasm as a soft tightening around our fingers, a sucking fish that hauled my whole body through her. She barely moved, but I bucked uncontrollably against his pelvic bone, rubbing and pushing as if I might tear through his body and into hers.

The boy rolled away and I wanted him to disappear, to leave us, me still reaching inside her, my fingers shaking and flexing and reaching, as if cracking the salty shell of an oyster and peeling back the flesh to find a pearl.

LOSING OUR JOBS

They told us to close the café early and I knew what was coming.

The atmosphere was funereal.

"Closing for refurbishment," they said and I felt my throat tightening. This was the end of it. All my workmates were my friends now. All the customers were ex-lovers or potential lovers or people I could wave to in the street.

"It's not about your work," they told us. "It's about profitability."

They let us go and we were never to come back. I knew that they did this so that we would not be tempted to lift packets of coffee or bottles of spirits on the way out.

We walked back from the city together and it struck me that we would not be able to afford next week's rent. I felt my face get hotter, and then wetter. Jessica wasn't crying. I wondered why I was crying when she wasn't. I would be handing in my thesis in a couple of months and the Austudy was almost over, and not nearly enough to cover the rent. I wondered about food.

"The universe will provide."

I wanted to tell her that the universe only provided for people who looked as pretty as she did and who had rich parents they could go home to if they really needed to, but it was all petty and nasty and it was no wonder she couldn't love me. No wonder I served as nothing but a distraction. I hunkered down into myself on that walk up the hill. I secured the hatches. I dried my tears on the night air and waved my resentment like a flag. Of course they would fire me. Of course I would have no money for rent. It was all destined to go wrong in the end.

By the time I reached the top of the hill, I was a small girl in the playground and my friends had abandoned me and they had taken my schoolbag and hidden it up in a tree but I wouldn't be budged. I would sit tight and silent and resentful.

She opened the door and put the Cocteau Twins on the record player. She poured me a vodka and put ice in it and a little blue plastic mermaid that she settled on the rim of the glass. There was, I knew, nothing to eat in the house. A packet of lentils in the cupboard that my grandmother had sent to us. "What are we going to do?" I asked, noticing the edge of stress in my voice. Jessica lay on the couch listening to her girly music. She rolled her eyes at my concern.

"I'll get some food. Write me a list."

She wrote the list for me because I imagined that she would prowl the supermarket in a big coat, slipping cans and packets into the various pockets. I had seen her take things before, not often, but I had seen it. I suppose there would be some leniency if we were only stealing a loaf of bread. Okay. Bread then, but she wrote sourdough and camembert and polenta and marinated olives. She made a note for coffee and for milk and cream. Cake, she wrote, chocolate, and because she knew that it was my favorite she wrote LINDT in capital letters beside this. She created a feast of eggplant and haloumi cheese and extra virgin olive oil on the back of an envelope.

I slumped onto the couch just as she bounced out of it.

She changed into a short silk skirt, her best bra with white flowers embroidered onto it, a low-cut shirt that showed off the bouquet in the places where it rested on the delicate curve of her breast. She headed out wearing lipstick and smelling like an ornamental garden in spring. Beautiful.

She returned with a man driving a red sports car. He was attractive, dressed in a casual but expensive suit. He was rich. I could smell it on him. He was holding four shopping bags in each hand. I suppose he was not used to lifting such a weight. I noticed his fingers trembling, but it was probably because she was standing in front of him in that short skirt and an obvious lack of underwear.

Groceries. Brie, olives, a nice white box containing a proper cake from a proper baker.

Her lipstick was perfect. She hadn't even kissed him. She didn't kiss him goodbye. She giggled. She allowed him to leave the bags on the front step and she waved as if he were already a long way away. I suppose he was.

THE INTERVIEW

It was a train then a bus then another bus. Then, at the end of this marathon of public transport, there was a climb, all dank-sock sweat and uphill trudge. I could see the beads of moisture forming on Jessica's forehead, bubbling up from under her makeup. Her lipstick should have been called open-wound red. Her mouth looked bloody and swollen. Vulnerable. I reached out and linked my fingers between Jessica's and her hand was slick with sweat. Our fingers slipped away from each other. A fat drip made a slow trail down my back and I felt it nestle between my buttocks.

"Should I have worn makeup?" I asked.

Jessica shrugged. She was still gorgeous. Her hair was wind-mussed, ripe with body heat and perfume. I hadn't worn perfume. I didn't own perfume, but I could have worn some of hers. I had never thought to use her techniques of seduction, her scents and her shampoos, her blush and her berry lipsticks. There on the hill, catching my breath in the dry-roast of suburban Runcorn, I began to wonder about that.

"You look fine," Jessica told me, by which she meant: you look sweaty and unkempt and not particularly feminine.

"We're almost there, aren't we?" Hopeful, staring up yet another hill, checking the map to see if there was an easier way around. There wasn't. We flapped the damp fabric of our shirts. A whiff of her perfume.

"Sweaty is fine," I told her. "Sweat is actually sexy."

We continued to climb.

I didn't know what we were expecting, but this wasn't it. The boy was too young, no more than twenty. He was wearing boardshorts and a Hawaiian shirt. No shoes. The flat was small and smelled faintly of mold. The carpet was threadbare in places and there were several empty XXXX cans crushed onto a breakfast bench dividing the lounge room from the kitchen. By the time I had stepped into his apartment I had decided that I didn't want the job but I had no way of communicating this to Jessica.

"We saw your ad in the paper," Jessica turned on the charm, a thick dollop of it, oozing out from under those heavy eyelids. Flirtation was her weapon. She aimed it expertly at the boy. I saw him waver under the onslaught. All his Christmases standing at his front door, with me as a distraction.

"Yes indeedee," he said. I glanced at the slight tenting of his boardshorts. "Glad you could come, ladies." Double entendre intended.

"How does this work?" Jessica asked, eyelashes stuttering low.

I had rarely heard her speak so many complete sentences in a row. I watched her working the situation and I bit my lip. We had made a mistake. I wanted to tell him up front and get it over with. We had made a mistake.

"Well," he was nervous. He scratched his elbow and I noticed a wide patch of scaly red where the skin was scraped raw. "After the audition, I just take bookings. Get this thing rolled out. How's that sound?"

Audition. The word fell with a hollow thud. It was the kind of word I remembered from undergrad, a word that sounded like panic attacks and had the acrid reek of phobia. Jessica was nodding.

"It's a double act," she cooed, her bedroom voice tickling his already attentive scrotum.

"All things are up for negotiation." He grinned. Leered.

She was nodding, but I was already shaking my head. I had my hand on her elbow, my fingers pressing into the soft skin. The audition was well and truly over.

At home in the lounge room, slipping off our shoes, I told her that I didn't want to work for the pimple-faced boy and she told me that she already knew it. I didn't really want to be a sex worker at all, even if it was just touching her with other people watching. She said that she had an audition at a strip club where she would wait on tables in her underwear.

"Make a cup of tea and bring it into my room?" she said to me.

I watched her slump off barefoot and heartbreakingly beautiful, up the stairs and into her bedroom.

Lying side by side without touching, I asked her if I smelled bad, like a wild animal, a bat, or a possum. She giggled and shifted so that her fragrant hair fanned out over her pillow the way I liked it.

"Don't be silly," she said, which wasn't really an answer.

"You only hold hands with me in public because you think that men find you more sexy if you're a lesbian," I said, not expecting an answer.

"You can sleep in here tonight. I don't mind. Go to sleep now," she said.

And eventually I did.

BRIAN AGAIN

Brian's car was parked out in front of our house and I found that I was angry. I wasn't sure how he'd found me, but Brisbane's a small town and someone told someone who told someone else and here was his car parked outside, a little askew, all of his bedding folded neatly on the back seat the way he liked it.

I wanted him to go away. I wanted to walk round the block once and come back and see that his car was gone. I thought about setting off, but it felt like the kind of pacing I associated with my dark times. Restless, a little off center. This was our house now. My house. I fitted the key in the lock and walked straight inside.

He was there at the table with her and she had one of her legs propped up on the edge of the chair and I could see she wasn't wearing underwear. Probably he could see that, too. She was laughing at something he had just said, giggling. Her flirtatious little laugh.

Have him. I thought, harshly, but I didn't think she would have him, really, not in that way. She didn't seem to sleep with anyone except her boyfriend unless she could pretend that they were sleeping with me and she was just close by, accidentally falling into the action, letting them worship at her flesh.

He turned when I entered the kitchen and I remembered his shiny eyes, all puppy-dog attention, the pretense of warmth.

"Back?" I asked him.

"It would seem so."

"How are you?"

"Thirsty."

I poured myself a vodka and put an olive into it. I felt like a martini but I knew we didn't have any vermouth. I measured the vodka left in the bottle against the light from the window—about an inch—and settled it back on the windowsill.

"I've brought a bottle of wine."

I nodded.

I wasn't going to drink his wine. I might if I finished the vodka, which seemed likely.

"Brian hasn't got anywhere to stay," Jessica told me. I already knew it.

"I said he could stay here if it's all right with you."

I thought about her boyfriend's brother; the man in the vacant lot who had wanted to sleep with her more than with me. I took a large sip of my vodka.

"If that's okay with you," he said to me. "I can sleep in my car if you like."

I shook my head.

"You can sleep in my room," I said.

I should have said no. I should have told him to sleep in his car. But if Jessica had told me to walk off a cliff I have no doubt I would have done it.

So he moved into my room, and I lost my skin. He slept with me that night and for many nights after and he listed my failings one by one.

"You still rely on that vibrator for an orgasm? The girls I like are fully in the moment. I'll teach you how to do it. Just be patient. Don't rush at sex like that. Women who are feminine know how to be patient, to wait, to time it. You know nothing about foreplay. Has anyone ever taught you about foreplay? Let me teach you about foreplay."

I watched him at the dinner table, entranced by her. I knew that he would trade beds in a second; I would, too. I still wanted her and I could see how obvious she was, how everybody wanted her.

I reveled in his ugliness. I made love to him and in my head I repeated, mantralike, "You are ugly and you are old and no one wants you except me and that makes me special."

I found a temporary gig at a restaurant but I was confused too easily. I miscounted tables, delivered the wrong meals to the wrong people. The bosses were kind to me but I knew I couldn't do the job effectively. Didn't want the job. I had to finish my thesis. I had to at least graduate from honors. I had to work out what I wanted to do with my life.

I had a key cut for him.

"One key," he said. "One key."

But by then I knew it was a line he had stolen from a movie and I made him take it anyway.

"I'll be up at the computer labs at uni," I told him. "You'll have to let yourself in."

"Jessica will let me in."

I didn't like him saying her name out loud.

"I'm still angry that you left last time without saying goodbye."

"You can't own a person," he said. "Everyone in the universe is free to move their energy where they please."

I knew then that he had been to the Living Game. He had been there with Jessica.

Sometimes at dinner I watched the two of them. Him watching her, her lowering her eyes shyly and giggling. I wondered if something had happened between them while I was in the computer lab. Perhaps at one of their sex seminars before he moved back in with me.

He went with me to a party. It was something a friend from university had organized, and although I rarely mixed my home life and my university life, I decided I would go and that I would bring him with me. We fought in the car on the way to the party. He closed his eyes and put his foot on the accelerator and said he would kill us then and there.

"For fuck's sake get it over with. Kill us, go on, kill us." He had been staying with me for weeks and it had begun to fall into a familiar pattern.

At the party, I sat in a corner and watched Brian making friends with all the beautiful girls from university. I knew I could never compete. I drank quietly by myself and when anyone came to sit with me I let them, and I nodded politely and answered in one-word sentences.

"I'm ready to go," I said at some point in the evening.

He had been flirting with a beautiful girl from the honors course, a girl I was quite fond of. He was filling her drink and engaging her in conversation. She was smart and sharp and they were deep in their banter.

"I'm not ready to go yet," he told me.

"All right. I'll walk home."

"All right," he said, although he knew it would take me an hour at least.

I liked walking in the dark. I liked the night. I liked the cool quiet of it. I liked the way the walking calmed me. I had been furious, I realized, as I turned into our own street. I wondered how long this anger had been percolating inside me. I was certain it had been longer than I would have admitted; I was furious still.

I can't afford this house, I thought as I walked toward it. Jessica made enough money dancing on tables and bending over groups of drunk men in her underwear with trays of overpriced drinks. I was flat out struggling with the rent every week. I spent hours at the markets, selling paintings I whipped up in minutes. I waited tables. I gathered my last few Austudy payments and waited for the day when I wouldn't be able to withdraw enough for my rent.

I let myself in quietly. Jessica was awake. I could hear her music drifting ethereally down the stairs. She might be alone; I could have climbed the stairs and said hello and made us a cup of tea, but these would not be the actions of a furious person. I slipped into my room and shut the door and lay down. There was no sleep anywhere. I stood up and I paced. It was eleven o'clock. I had left the party just before ten. I wondered what Brian would be doing. I wondered what Brian had done. Specifically I wondered what Brian had done with Jessica. If she had done anything with him it would be because he wanted her and because he was sleeping with me. I imagined that she wanted to prove that she could win in everything. I remembered her thing with her boyfriend's brother and no matter what I had done, I would never do that.

I heard his car at three in the morning. I had been pacing, painting, reading, pacing some more. I left the apartment briefly and set out for a walk, realized it would be pointless, and let myself back in again. I dressed and undressed and dressed and undressed.

I settled on a T-shirt and sat at the canvas, making white fingerprints on it. I didn't like the image that was emerging, a woman, shrouded in what looked like bandages, seen from above, mostly white, a light shading of blue, the eyes upward gazing and rimmed in red.

I looked at the painting and knew I was still furious.

When I heard his car I leaped into bed and rolled onto my side. I might have been asleep.

He removed his shoes. He removed his socks. He removed his clothes, and the sag of his body shuffled into bed beside me. He warmed his hands on my hips.

"I like your friends," he said. "They are fun."

I wanted to pretend that I was still sleeping, but I was a fist and he could feel the tension in my body and so I rolled onto my back and stared up at the ceiling. "You think they are beautiful."

"Yes."

"More beautiful than me."

"Yes. All of them are so much more beautiful than you." Here came the list. I rolled my eyes as he began it. "More warm. More feminine. More giving. More compassionate. More understanding."

He rolled onto me then, he was hard, but I didn't want to. I wanted him to go back to the party. I wanted him to sleep with all the beautiful women who were more beautiful than me. I was angry because I knew it was true and I hated him for saying it.

"I don't," I said. "I don't want to do this."

But he wanted to. He held my hands in his fist and he raised them above my head and I tried to slip out from under him but he was heavy and I had no skin left at all. It might be easier to let him do it, I thought. Get it over with. After all, I had never said no to sex before. I tried to remove my hands from his fists and it seemed to be his weight that pinned me but of course it wasn't. I was powerless because he told me with each thrust that I was hideous, and with each thrust I believed him.

"I'd be fucking her if I could," he said. "You are nothing in comparison. Easy ride. Not the same class of woman."

And I found myself unable to argue, unable to struggle my hands out from the place where he held them above my head. I wondered what had once held me together, because now I was dispersing, falling into pieces on the bed.

I had never said no. This is what I came to when he pushed himself inside me and made the angry thrusts with his hips. I could hear him talking. I knew the list was continuing. I was not the girlfriend kind, I was less than all of them in very fundamental ways. And I agreed with him. I completely agreed with him, but I was focused on the sudden realization that I had never ever said no to anyone. The other girls, the girlfriend kind of girls, they all said no at one time or another.

I refocused my eyes. He was sweating over me. He was red faced. He might have had a heart attack from the effort it took to have sex with me when I refused to cooperate.

"No," I tried out the word. He did not hear me. "No. Stop. I want you to stop."

He hadn't paused to put on a condom. He knew I wouldn't have sex without a condom and here he was, ejaculating into me without one.

He rolled off me. He was still angry, I could tell, but it was tempered now by the exhaustion that follows climax.

I could feel the sticky juices of him dripping out of me. I would have to get the morning after pill. I thought this and I remembered my first time. My very first time. All the blood and pain and negotiation.

"I didn't like that," I said, and he said nothing, but I knew he had heard me. "I didn't like that at all."

I rolled over and I felt the sticky mess of him dripping out of me, staining the sheets. The morning after pill would make me sick. I had vomited last time. I had been sick as a dog for hours after. It felt like the flu. I closed my eyes, stepping through the trip I would make to the doctor in the morning, the interminable wait in the foyer with all the sick and dying people. I should get tested for STDs, too, although I would have to wait three months to find out what I had picked up from this evening's entertainment. I thought all of this through, dispassionately, and although I thought I might never sleep it was midmorning when I found myself awake again.

He bought me a dozen red roses and told me he had never bought anybody flowers before, and I thanked him for it. This terrible double-crossing of myself. This is what I regret more than anything.

He left in the middle of the night when I wasn't expecting it. I woke up and he was gone, and I started to cry although I was sure I must be happy that he was gone. I cried for the whole day, rocking back and forth, his list playing on a loop in my head. I am ugly. I am crass. I am coarse. I am unfeminine. I am too harsh. I am too honest. I have no secrets. I am too obvious. I am too sexual. I am too aggressively sexual. I am like a man. I am not like a girlfriend. I am unlovable. I am. I am. I am.

MANTRA

Brisbane 2008

I am ugly. I am crass. I am coarse. I am unfeminine. I am too harsh. I am too honest. I have no secrets. I am too obvious. I am too sexual. I am too aggressively sexual. I am like a man. I am not like a girlfriend. I am unlovable. I am ugly. I am crass. I am coarse. I am unfeminine. I am too harsh. I am too honest. I have no secrets. I am too obvious. I am too sexual. I am too aggressively sexual. I am like a man. I am not like a girlfriend. I am unlovable. I am ugly. I am crass. I am coarse. I am unfeminine. I am too harsh. I am too honest. I have no secrets. I am too obvious. I am too sexual. I am too aggressively sexual. I am like a man. I am not like a girlfriend. I am unlovable. I am. I am. I am. I am I am I am I am I am I am I am I am I am I am I am I am I am I am I am I am I am I.

BALLOONS

Brisbane 1990

Jessica held my head in her lap and told me to breathe deeply. People were running inside my chest, big men, hurdling, running and jumping and thumping down on my ribs. I was filled with athletes and my arms were locked and rigid over my chest. She told me to breathe and I managed a halting breath that was half a sob and I smelled her secret musky odor under the sweet floral perfume. It made me even more agitated.

I was the gnarled and gnomic Rumpelstiltskin from the fairytale. I was all spit and struggle. She was a part of the problem offering a solution. She kissed my tears and I could love her or I could hit her; I was bouncing from one state to the next like someone leaping from rock to rock in an ice-capped stream.

"Imagine," she told me, "that for every breath there is a balloon filling."

Balloons. She had learned that trick in one of her self-help sessions. I felt my chest tightening. I had lived with her affirmations pinned to the wall in the toilet, tolerating her self-deluding platitudes for the sake of her extraordinary beauty. Now she hugged me and I struggled away from her.

"Release the balloons," she whispered. "One by one." Someone else's words from her ripe, overblown mouth. The mouth I had bitten. The mouth that I had pressed my nipple against, that had never sullied itself against my vagina. Her perfect mouth.

The balloons slipped from my fingers one by one.

When they were gone, floating off into the angry pale of the sky, there was nothing left for me to hold onto.

I rolled out of her empty hug and I was gone. I had already left the room.

"That's right," she told me. "Let go of the balloons, one by one by one."

One by one by one and it was all gone. I was gone. She was gone. There was nothing left to hold onto and my chest eased out of the vice that had gripped it. I left the room. I left the house. I left that life. And I was gone.

THE LONGING

Brisbane 2008

I am buffeted between conflicting states. I am at once wrung out by longing, swelling like dough under a damp cloth into the idea of Paul. It is a strange alchemy that blends smell and flesh into some pheromonal melting pot. I harbor secret glimpses of possible outcomes, which inevitably include climbing into his lap and settling into the hardness there. I imagine hand-holding in libraries or lying on the grass or in the cinema. These random images are thrown up at inappropriate moments, in company, on the bus, at work. I catch my breath so it won't escape in a moan or a little sigh.

It is not the first time I have had this kind of all-consuming crush on someone who is not my husband. It crashes in, and it abates. I am used to the pattern. It is a pattern but I am still surprised by the force of the desire.

At the same time there is a rock solid care for Paul, a familial love, the kind that you would imagine a big sister would have for a beloved brother. I would fight for him, scuff my knees. If he called in the middle of the night he would find me at his side without any subtext. Still, I would eat him if I could. I would carve through his flesh with a spoon and gorge myself on him.

I turn in on myself, wondering what I might do to elicit the same kind of passion from him. And even as I conjure up possibilities, I know. I am not blind. He will never want me. There is my physicality, my age, my erratic nature. I would remake myself into someone else to catch his attention. I wonder if he would love a thinner girl. That pretty blond thing I saw him with, the sunken eyes and skin that looked as if you would bruise it with a glance. I would carve myself up into pieces to have him look at me that way. I would stop eating. I would learn to wear makeup and perfume like a real girl.

PARK
Brisbane 1990

When I stopped running I was in a park. Light fell like snow onto the grass. Solid light. This is what I noticed first, the painterly quality of the light. The park was beautiful. The trees were solid patches of darkness. I had somehow run myself out of the world and here I was in a painting by Edward Hopper, an in-between place of flat shapes and silence and all the panic drained out and dissipated. It was a perfect summer evening. My eyes were still red and sore from weeping. My chest was still tight. Behind me was the memory of a storm, not a gentle storm, but the kind that rips the roof off a house and flings cars into a flooded street. Sirens, screaming, bodies ripped from the hands of lovers and raced away into the turmoil of a drowning.

I sat on one of the well-lit benches and there was a downy light in my lap. I had picked up my satchel before running: I had a book and a pad of cartridge paper and my little box of pastels and a pen. Everything I needed, for a while at least. I was a small vessel and I could bob here in the calm waters until some other vessel came along.

I sat until the shrieking in my head had settled. I sipped the silence and felt myself relax into the void. I could stay here, of course, calcifying moment by slow moment. I could spend the rest of my life sitting in glorious silence on this very bench.

I thought about sex. If I were to live here forever on this bench in this park that might have been painted by Hopper, I would need to find somewhere else to have sex.

I had had sex in this park. I glanced around me and found the spot, a place near a tree, on a scratchy bed of leaves. My body remembered the crackle of them, the thrill of air on my thighs as the boy flipped up my long skirt and slipped inside me just as quickly. The small half-hearted tussle between him and me. The shrugging into sex despite the fact that it was daylight and there were offices and people readying themselves to spill out from their air-conditioned comfort and into this very park. It was quick and kind of fun although I didn't really like him very much. And I didn't orgasm. I remembered that.

So, yes, I could in fact have sex in this park, or in the toilet block or in the shrubbery hugging the fence a little way from my bench. In fact the shrubbery could be a place to sleep, I suspected, all snuggled and scrubby and safe through the balmy Brisbane nights. I could sleep in the comfort of crawl spaces, under shrubs, in cupboards, hidden under a bed. This was my preferred sleeping option actually. A water fountain, too. There was one just near to me. All the comforts of a house without the rigid trap of walls to bounce off. No roommates to watch and judge me. No Jessica and no Brian. No address to be found at, just a series of comforting spaces with grass and trees and the scent of night jasmine and all this blissful silence.

I looked around me now as if I were inspecting a property that I might purchase. Yes, I thought. I could just stay here.

THE TOILET BLOCK

The boy sat on the bench, waiting. He positioned himself under a light, in full view. I viewed him there, sleek and pale, furtive, but with a sudden calm descending when someone came by. I was hidden under a hedge, pressed between the woody scramble of it, against a wire fence. I had a coat wrapped around me and a satchel for a pillow.

Everywhere the insect rustling of leaves, a balmy, cockroachy, Brisbane summer kind of night and me out in it. I was black on black and he was all golden glow.

There was the toilet block nearby. This is how it seemed to work. One boy, this golden boy, would sit, jiggling his knee till some other boy arrived. This one was a dark shadow, edging by his arc of park-light. The new man waited outside the toilet block for a while, pacing idly as if he were just filling in time before popping back to work.

Then the deliberate stride into the squat brick building, a significant pause. The golden boy now still and upright, tight inside his pale clothing, erect, straining up from his seat as if he were a volcanic eruption about to occur.

When he stood he was like a soldier on parade. All the straight-armed tension in his body turning stride into march. I watched him glance around stiffly, checking. How long does it take to get a head job in a toilet block? Or was there more to it? Was there a partial removal of clothing, a bare-backed fucking, one knee braced on the toilet seat? I imagined the golden boy bent over the cistern in that sickly blue light they use to thwart junkies looking for a vein.

The thing about homelessness is that there is nowhere comfortable and private for masturbation. I clamped my hand between my legs and nestled my pubic bone against it. I rubbed quickly. No one would notice me down here in the dark crawl space under a hedge. No one would expect a human being to settle down for the night in a claustrophobic place like this.

The boys took significantly longer than I did. I watched, smoothing my skirt down over my drawn-up knees as another, older man crept into the spotlight and nestled down in the waiting space.

I wondered what would happen if I needed to use the toilet. Would I be holding up the queue? I closed my eyes, dozed, opened them. A new man sitting, smoking, waiting. I felt the throb in my bladder, but if I just held on I knew it would pass.

There was no panic. That was the strangest thing. For the first time in so long I was calm. Perhaps I was happy. Perhaps I was invisible. When someone caught sight of me they looked away quickly enough; their gaze didn't stick.

I still walked but it was different, no longer the kind of walking that was almost a chase. I was not outwalking something that frightened me. I barely looked around to see if anything was chasing me. There was the breeze on my skin. Sharp scents. The colors were heightened, like the times I had tried LSD. There was some sleep, taken in small doses. At all other times there was sound and movement and color and I was happy, perhaps ecstatic. I knew that I couldn't live like this forever. I knew that I must come to some kind of resolution, but for now I was completely content.

I was floating down the hill toward the city when a small girl turned around and suddenly my invisibility was shattered. Her eyes narrowed as she spotted me and she tugged at her mother's arm.

"Mummy."

"What?"

"Mummy."

Her mother glanced in the direction of her pointing finger.

"Look at that lady."

Her mother looked at me then quickly away. She shushed her child and I heard her whispered words. "Don't stare at her."

Me. Don't stare at me.

In the city I glanced at my reflection in a hundred glass windows. My clothes, my face, my eyes.

And I knew suddenly why I was no longer frightened for myself. I had become the person people are frightened of. I had slipped somehow from the inside to the outside of everything. And there I stood, staring at them through the window of a department store.

I have left, I thought to myself. Finally after all of these years of trying, I have actually left the world.

I walked though the streets of Brisbane and I remembered and I felt a longing. There had been no one touching my skin for almost a month. No physical interaction, no conversation. No people.

I practiced remembering. The couch. The one that felt like velvet and had to be sponged afterward because it stained. The sisal carpet, the one with the rope burns. In the cupboard, where I had felt the safest, despite the limited opportunities for movement. On the balcony, and only because of the drugs and the hour of the morning. On the boardwalk in the botanical gardens where we could pretend I was just sitting on his lap. In the archbishop's garden, and only because I couldn't see the fascination she had with it. In the bus stop because the bus was delayed. On the train because the train was delayed. In the restaurant because the food was delayed. In the kitchen because of the implements. In the garden because of the dirt. In the bath because of the lack of dirt. In the bed. Sometimes, even in the bed.

I would shift back on the park bench and expect to feel the hardness of a penis behind me. I watched two birds fall onto each other, a raised twitchy tail and I could feel it, this slipping inside each other, when was the last time I was held, really held and for no other reason than for pleasure?

The birds parted. Wrens. They were wrens. I was almost certain of it. Their coupling had been cute and quick and bouncy. I wanted that kind of sudden sex. I wanted to participate in it, not watch it from the sidelines. But most of all I wanted, suddenly, just to be held.

NIGHTMARE

Brisbane 2008

In my dream. The thin girl is trying to break in through the window at the back of the house. She is myself, only starved and hungry. She is looking for somebody else to fill her. She frightens me, all wild hair and mouth like a boiling kettle, and I push my shoulder against the window until she is gone. The sudden relief of her absence. I rest against the wall. I catch my breath. My dream self realizes suddenly that the front door has been left wide open. She is inside.

I close my eyes in horror and I wake. She is inside. She is with me now, even as I lie in the sweat and the shivering of my bed. She is all the things that have been said to me. She is not the girlfriend kind of girl, and yet I roll over and I touch the warm shoulder of my husband, my beautiful lover who smiles in his sleep, remembering that I am here and that I love him.

I read back over my life. I see myself lying in the wonderfully suggestible place between orgasms. Some body or another in contact with my own. I hear their voices drifting with me into sleep. Not my type. Not the girlfriend type. So many repetitions on a theme. I ingest their words, I am soft and open in the afterglow and I take this into myself. The words exit my skin like splinters of glass working their way out of me over the course of years.

I roll over and I hold him, my husband.

"I had a nightmare," I whisper and he snuggles back against me sleepily.

"Poor darling," he says, and "I love you," and "You're beautiful."

RAIN
Brisbane 1991

I was sitting in a doorway, not a particularly large doorway, not a comfortable one, but it was free from vomit despite a distant urinous stench emanating from the far corners. I had a quarter bottle of scotch. Scotch was not my drink of choice, but it was cheap, and they didn't have any small bottles of vodka, and the day was cold.

The man at the shop gave it to me in a paper bag and I folded the top of the bag down with the bottle inside, as if no one would know that I was sitting in a doorway drinking a quarter bottle of scotch if I hid the label.

The man at the bottle shop nodded toward the window, acknowledging the rain falling, quick and loud.

"Lovely weather," he said to make conversation. I was supposed to say something back, perhaps something witty, something to augment his little joke. But I had spoken to no one in so many days. I felt my heart spring in my chest, a small animal inside me attempting to scramble away from the nice bottle shop man. I blinked and struggled with my expression. I said nothing, handed the coins across the counter, took the brown paper bag.

The rain came down like this sometimes. It was a tropical phenomenon, this drenching in the heart of summer, tearing the breathless heat apart and hinting at the possibility of ice.

In the past I would watch the occasional downpour from my window, or run out into it and race back into a hot shower and dry clothes, laughing with the manic energy induced by sudden storms.

Now there would be no shower. Now there would be wet shoes and a slow iciness creeping into my bones. Now there would be nothing but shivering and feeling sorry for myself. I didn't want to cry but thinking about not crying made my shoulders heave. I took another swig from the bottle.

I was sitting in a doorway drinking scotch from a paper bag. It was raining. My skirt smelled old and damp. The pages of my notebook would be curling. My beetling words inside the notebook would be bleeding onto the page. There was a night ahead of me and another day and another night and more again and the idea of it exhausted me.

"I've got to find a place," I said the words out loud. I found that I did that a lot. The lack of communication had somehow changed my relationship to speech. Sometimes a word would slip out of my mouth.

Sometimes a whole sentence. Sometimes I caught myself in the middle of an entire conversation, questions and answers, a heated sparring with myself.

"I'm going mad," I told myself, tucking my shoes up a step and out of the back spray of rain. "I am talking to myself," I said to myself. "And I have to get out of the rain."

THE DEPARTMENT
OF SOCIAL SECURITY

There is a bleakness common to all government buildings. The mood-affecting color schemes; posters, a repetition of warnings we will read but not heed. I stared at an antismoking poster and considered ducking outside for a cigarette. A safe-sex poster and I thought about unprotected sex. Alcohol, violence. I had been waiting for over an hour and a grim cocktail was percolating inside me. The music didn't help. It was tragic radio. Not the kind of radio I would choose to listen to, but the fug of sound that is chosen for its inability to offend. I was, of course, offended by the gray carpet of music, not to mention the actual gray carpet which seemed to have cigarette burns in it despite the no-smoking signs. I still felt like a cigarette. I glanced at a poster for domestic violence and wondered if I would kill for one.

When they called my name I was twitchy as a junky. I had knotted the end of my skirt and it dragged high against my calf. There were little balls of paper, torn corners from a magazine, a little pyramid of them piled next to my chair. I didn't remember doing this, but I recognized the architecture constructed by my own restless fingers. My calling card, this miniature nest like something a bowerbird might construct.

I gathered my things. Papers, pens, my satchel. Things fell from my bag that I didn't know I had, seedpods, cigarette papers—a brand I'd never heard of. I felt I had been sleepwalking, gleaning the detritus of the world without consciousness.

When I had collected the various bits and pieces of my life I scurried toward the counter. The man, boy, he was no more than a boy, looked at me. I saw him sniff. I wondered if my clothes had started to smell like a homeless person; that nasty mix of scalp and urine and cigarette smoke that we draw away from when we encounter it on public transport.

I had not spoken for many days. When he asked if he could help me his words were loud and pointed. Could he help me? I wondered if he could. I wondered if it would be possible to help me. This seemed suddenly like so huge a question I could barely find a sentence to begin the interaction.

"I have no money."

I swayed back in my chair, overwhelmed by the initiation of what must inevitably become a conversation.

"You're unemployed?"

I nodded. He was waiting for more and so I dragged myself forward in my chair. "I lost my job," I told him and he nodded, making notes.

"When did you become unemployed?"

I counted back. Not so long ago but it seemed like a lifetime.

"Maybe three months ago."

"Savings?"

I shook my head.

"Address?"

I shook my head.

"You don't have an address? Where have you been living?"

I shrugged and leaned back in the hard plastic chair, "Nowhere in particular."

Such a complicated conversation. I was exhausted by it. Behind me there was a woman with a child that had begun to wind up into that terrible shrieking only children can manage. Outside men with tattoos on their necks dragged frantically on cigarettes clutched in the shelter of their fists. Military-style smoking; or prison. A man in the corner of the room was rocking ever so slightly backwards and forwards. His lips twitched to a barely contained inner monologue.

"Are you homeless?"

I looked back toward the boy and he seemed suddenly concerned. Was I homeless? I had no place to be in particular, but what does that mean exactly?

"Maybe. I suppose so."

"Where have you been sleeping?"

I thought about the crawl space behind the bushes in Albert Park. I thought about Laura's empty house, while she was at work, her leather couch and the little stretch of grass at the side of her pool. I thought about the place at Highgate Hill where you could see the whole world. If you lay there for long enough little purple flowers puddled in your clothing. I felt like I should tell him all of this, because the bare truth of it sounded harsh. I scuffed my Docs against the threadbare gray carpet.

"In a park mostly," I told him and it sounded melodramatic. Homeless girl, living in a park. I wanted to tell him that I had no money but never drank instant coffee. I wanted to explain about my afternoons in the cinema with the free choc-tops and the free broken quiches from Aromas. I wanted to point to the man who had stopped rocking and who was standing now, his lips forming silent words. In the scheme of things, I wanted to say, I was coddled.

He pressed a form into my hand.

"Fill in as much of this as you can and bring it straight back to the counter," he told me. I took his form and the pen he handed to me and I stood without explaining myself at all.

I read the questions. Name, date of birth, address. I needed a cigarette. I held the pen in my fist, struggled to remember the correct spelling of my name.

I needed a cigarette and sex and alcohol. I needed to be somewhere

where there was sun and wind and little purple flowers. I needed to be somewhere where the tears that had begun to obscure my vision could fall neatly into the dirt and grass where they would be gone and no one would see them.

Name. Krissy Kneen. Kris, really, but everyone called me Krissy, and Kneen was not the name I was born with but it was my grandfather's name and that was fine. I could choose to use my father's name instead, or my grandmother's because it was my grandmother I longed for when I had a headache or when I was lonely. My grandmother who would say, "There is no try, only do or do not do," like some ancient Eastern European Yoda figure. My grandmother who would say, "Don't be silly, you are not homeless at all. You are in between your houses," as if I would rummage and find a key in the bottom of my bag along with the stones and seeds and poetry-laden scraps of paper.

What is the current balance of your bank account? "You are not broke," my grandmother's voice told me. She was in my head. She watched through my eyes as I wrote $4.00 and she was shaking her head. "Not broke, fashionably fancy free."

Broke. I answered her back and I should never answer her back. She would never tolerate this kind of disrespect. Broke and homeless and in need of some assistance. Some help. I tipped my head forward so that the tears bypassed my cheeks and fell neatly onto the page. When my eyes were dry I saw the saltwater had smudged the form.

My last name could be Kneen or Knoon; even Know. I blotted the page with my sleeve and blew on it till it was dry. I carefully filled in the double "e." Kneen. Kris Kneen. I brushed the surface of the page clean and continued to fill in the form.

CHAPTER FORTY

Brisbane 2008

Beauty is all about symmetry, they say. Some perfect form of balance. My own eye seems to slide off the things that others consider beautiful. Symmetry does not capture my attention; I am more drawn to the person who feels misplaced. The loners, the overlooked, the undervalued. I like my houses tumbledown and my bookshelves a patchwork of spines at a lean.

Perhaps it should be no surprise to me, then, that I woke up this morning and found that I was beautiful. Not pretty. Not like the girls who turn heads and who earn free cocktails just by bestowing their symmetry on others. Not like Jessica or even Laura or Katherine or any of those girls I have wanted or wanted to become. I woke, and did not need to look in a mirror to know that somehow I had overlooked the obvious.

I am my own tumbledown building. I am the joyful expanse of my own flesh with the marks of age and a life of pleasure worn proudly like any graffiti-strewn alley. I like my own taste, admire it even. I like who I am. I am strangely surprised by this. I like what my body does when I am touching it. I like the skill with which I bring myself to orgasm. I like the way I orgasm, contained and yet abandoned to the pleasure of it. I like that I can find pleasure in the slightest disturbance of the air.

I like myself. How could this be? I barely recognize my relationship to myself. Gone is the stress and worry, my constant assessing and reassessing of my own behavior. I try on clothes and face a mirror fearlessly for perhaps the first time in my life. I am short and large and odd looking. My face is not pretty and my body is certainly not something to be reproduced endlessly like a photograph of a model or a parade of catwalk beauties each one so similar to the next. I am myself and I am beautiful in my own very particular way. This self-liking makes me uneasy, but I am fine with that as well. It is the kind of uneasiness that I can love.

So I walk past the Story Bridge and there is my iPod and the Pixies, and I pick the kind of grass with the gray pink tufts that I love so much and there is the Story Bridge that I think perhaps I might jump off, but I know probably I won't. I listen to the Pixies and I think I might listen to the Pixies again tomorrow, on my fortieth birthday.

Instantly and overnight it is different. This is how the change has occurred. I am new in my skin. I am a quiet strength. I have been clinging to my younger self like a life jacket, comforted by the whistle and the toggles and the little light. For a moment that lasted twenty years I had forgotten about my own natural buoyancy. Now that the fall is behind me I can feel the pleasure of the slap of waves and the little nipping of fish that share the water with me. I know about sharks that lurk and the possible dangers they bring with them, but I am a wily creature. I look back on my life so far and I know that it is true. I have swum through hoops, slick as a dolphin, and all this play has been good training for my sudden transition. From the paddling pool to the lap pool—and now this high-diving act has brought me to the ocean. The dangerous, glorious ocean, replete with the possibility of whales.

ST. JAMES STREET

Brisbane 1990

I could live there. This small room with its single bed. A single bed. I thought I could perhaps drag my king-size futon from under Laura's house and lay it out on all the available floor space. The edge of it would butt up against the sink but I could be careful with my washing up. Or I could roll the futon up during the day, or I could stick with the single bed. A single bed and the celibacy it implied.

A man shuffled out into the corridor to stare at me. They were all men. I could smell them, the horror of unwashed socks and stained underwear, old-man's long johns hidden under flannel shirts. The man was older than me, but not so old. Maybe in his fifties, probably not too much older than Brian. I clutched my bag, suddenly aware of the low swing of my shirt and my breasts swelling out of it. The man stared with the kind of unabashed curiosity that we must grow into, all shyness abandoned after hard years of practice. I stepped back into the room that might be mine. A sink, a bed, a tiny desk, a stove and an oven that may or may not have worked. It was affordable and I could live there.

The caretaker shook his head at me.

"I won't rent it to you."

I watched the old man shuffle back into his room. The door rattled closed. Loose paint flaked onto the musty carpet. He would be my neighbor. At night I might hear his pathetic attempts at masturbation. We would share the shower down the hallway. I would find his gray pubic hairs fossilized in the communal soap.

"I can afford it."

"I won't." He swept his arm across the shadowy view of the corridor with its myriad of closed doors. "Old alcoholic men. That's who live here. And junkies. I'm not renting it to you."

I took a step back and the floorboards creaked. Outside the clouds were gathering. It would rain again.

He walked me to the front steps. "It's not for you," he told me, concerned. "Look love," and I could have hit him; my hand became a fist, the nails bit into my palm, "there."

He pointed out toward the overcast sky. I squinted but I couldn't see anything—just a hill I would have to walk up and houses pressed hip to hip; coming rain.

"Up at the top, near the Fiveways, there's a block of apartments. Cheap. I know there's a couple free. You should check that out."

"I've got the deposit," I told him. "I've got it in cash."

He eased me down the stairs, the flat of his palm in my back. "St. James Street," he told me. "I don't know the number."

Rain spat in my face when I glanced upward. Light rain, but it would get heavier. I breathed in jasmine. Exhaled gardenia. It was a Brisbane summer day and there was rain coming.

There were angels in the garden. White stone creatures perched on dry fountains. There were naked women hoisting stone basins onto their shoulders. There was a house behind these whitewashed figures. The house was perched at a lean, heavier on its top floor than it was below. Threatening to spill bathrooms and lounge rooms down into the weedy garden with its picket fence.

I climbed crumbling steps and knew as soon as I stepped up onto the tumbledown porch that I would live there. A blue heeler lifted its lazy head from its paws, its eyebrows crinkling over sleepy eyes. I smiled and bent and patted its solid head and I smelled its doggy scent on my fingers. This was the room, the one that the dog was guarding.

Beside the dog was a broken couch with a blanket thrown over its spilled stuffing. There was a man asleep on the couch. He was all elbows and knees and his breath caught in a discreet snore that sounded more like the purr of a contented cat. There was paint on his fingers, red paint. There was paint on his shirt and I noticed his sandals were an abstract work of red and yellow splatters. He smelled like my family. Turpentine, linseed oil, nicotine. His fingers had the yellow stains of a heavy smoker. There was a pouch of tobacco on the couch beside him. Dr. Pat. The same tobacco that I had been smoking. The same tobacco my grandfather used in his pipe.

I was careful not to wake him as I stepped over the dog and slipped the key into the door.

There were two rooms inside. The first was nothing more than a large bay window but it was big enough for my bed and the view was fringed by frangipani flowers and bougainvillea. The floorboards were already dripped with a splatter from the haphazard paint job. The kitchen sink was half aluminum, half rust. No toilet, somewhere there would be a shared toilet and a shower, but there was a gas stovetop and a bar heater on the wall. I would be fed and I would be warm. I suspected I would be happy.

I stepped out onto the porch and the young man was awake and leaning on one hand as he rolled a cigarette with another. He blinked, squinted. He pushed himself up until he was sitting a little unsteadily. There was an odd, unfocused vagueness in his eyes, but he looked straight at me and he grinned as if we were great friends.

"Ah," he said to me. "You're home then."

SEX, LOVE, AND INTIMACY

Brisbane 2008

Of course Paul will leave with this girl. Paul is single and she is pretty and we did not arrive together. There is no reason for him to be anywhere but here, leaning across this dirty café table scorching this young girl in the blaze of his attention. He is charming; I have been charmed. Now it is her turn to be flattered into adoration. He will leave with her, and our other friends will sidle up to their temporary partners and drift off into the dawn.

It is one in the morning and drizzling. Our apartment is less than an hour's walk away.

I stand and leave the table unnoticed. The rain comes harder when I am at the first set of traffic lights, rivulets finding the contours of my cheeks. No one has seen me leave. This is a game; teams have been selected and I am here at the edge of things, watching for a while, leaving, finding my way home.

At the venue there were bands and I felt like dancing but they don't seem to dance anymore, this younger cooler generation. A night of sitting quietly in corners, everyone so young and self-aware and beautiful.

The rain is heavier the farther I trudge toward home. My dress clings to my body. The night is reflected in sad, damp puddles that lick at the edges of my shoes.

This is why married women who are forty do not go out to see bands with friends half their age. First there is the odd conversation with the Indian cab driver about the disposal of corpses in which somehow, in the time it takes to slide between one suburb and another, my body shape is likened to that of both a seal and a dugong. Then there is the line-up at the door where everyone is carded except me. Then there is the fact that I have more income than my student friends and it seems morally wrong to let them buy me a drink even though I have already bought them one or two. Then there is this pairing off, this settling into coupledom that will leave me walking home in the rain when they are all settling into cabs, snuggling up beside each other warm and dry in the hug of intimacy.

Inside my quiet apartment the calm takes me by surprise. The chaos of my day-to-day existence has been cleared away. Books shelved, benches wiped, dishes washed and neatly stacked. The sound of the rain is a gentle lullaby. I have drunk too much but I am not reeling drunk. I am wet but not chilled to the bone, and there in my bed is my own prize. The boy I would have left with if I had met him at the bar—even now, in our harried middle age. I look at his sleeping face and know that I would have spotted him immediately, found some way to share a cab with him or entice him out into the rain.

I peel off my soaked clothing and towel myself dry in the darkness of the bathroom. Our bathroom. Our house. When I slip into our bed he nestles sleepily against me.

"Hello Beautiful." A dreamy whisper.

"Hi there."

"It's raining."

"I walked home in the rain."

"You should have caught a cab."

"No," I tell him and I touch his dry hair, curling my fingers through it gently. "It was nice, walking in the rain. Like I used to do."

"How are your little friends?" he asks me, waking a little, grinning.

"Cute," I tell him. "But you are so much cuter."

"I know," he grins and closes his eyes and shuffles closer. "And I know you know it, too."

"I do. Please never forget that I do."

I settle next to him. I smell the wonderful warm scent of him, knowing that this will not be the last time I wander home, tipsy and wet and alone; abandoned by all my exciting young friends. Knowing also that my husband will be here for me, sleepy, dry, waiting. The man who I once picked out of a crowd, and who I would pick again and again if I were meeting him anew.

ABOUT THE AUTHOR

Krissy Kneen is a writer and bookseller. She has written short films and directed documentaries for Australian television. She is the author of a short collection of erotica, *Swallow the Sound,* and she lives in Brisbane, Australia, with her husband. *Affection* is her first book.

ACKNOWLEDGMENTS

My writer and bookseller friends are the most supportive people that I know. They have stood by me for so many years and my joy with this book is theirs to share.

In particular I thank: Chris Somerville, Christopher Currie, Katherine Lyall-Watson, Fiona Stager, Nike Bourke, Benjamin Law, Kristina Olsson, Nick Earls, Angela Meyer, Kirsten Reed, Trent Jamieson, Ronnie Scott. Thanks to the crew at QWC and particularly to Kate Eltham. Also to the ever-tolerant team at Avid Reader Bookshop and Café who fed me scotch when I was crying and champagne when I was elated during the writing of this book.

I would also like to thank my family, Wendy, Lotty, Barry, Karen, Peter R., Sheila, Denise, Helen and Peter M.

Thank you also to the friends and lovers who were there with me through my wild days. A special thanks to Elissa Freeman and Bec Harbison: twin pillars of support, and Judith Lukin-Amundsen, a most marvelous mentor.

The biggest thanks to Mandy Brett for the most amazing edit (a tighter, leaner, stronger book because of you), and to the team at Text Publishing. I stand in awe.

Selected Titles from Seal Press

For more than thirty years, Seal Press has published groundbreaking books. By women. For women. Visit our website at www.sealpress. com. Check out the Seal Press blog at www.sealpress.com/blog.

Good Porn: A Woman's Guide, by Erika Lust. $17.95, 978-1-58005-306-8. Fun, fact-filled, and totally racy, *Good Porn* is an unapologetic celebration of porn—and a guide both for women who like it and those who don't know what they're missing.

Dirty Girls: Erotica for Women, edited by Rachel Kramer Bussel. $15.95, 978-1-58005-251-1. A collection of tantalizing and steamy stories compiled by prolific erotica writer Rachel Kramer Bussel.

Free Fall: A Late-in-Life Love Affair, by Rae Padilla Francoeur. $16.95, 978-1-58005-304-4. In this erotic memoir, Rae Padilla Francoeur recounts the joys, benefits, and challenges of embarking upon a surprising love affair late in life, and inspires women over 50 to discover their deepest sexual self.

Sex and Bacon: Why I Love Things That Are Very, Very Bad for Me, by Sarah Katherine Lewis. $14.95, 978-1-58005-228-3. A sensual—and sometimes raunchy—book celebrating the intersection of sex and food.

Fucking Daphne: Mostly True Stories and Fictions, edited by Daphne Gottlieb. $15.95, 978-1-58005-235-1. An erotic collection of stories—all centered on the fictional character "Daphne"—that blurs the line between fact and fantasy.

Sweet Charlotte's Seventh Mistake, Cori Crooks. $18.95, 978-1-58005-249-8. In this stunning visual memoir, Cori Crooks searches for her identity among the old photographs, diary entries, and letters left behind by her delinquent family.

Find Seal Press Online

www.SealPress.com
www.Facebook.com/SealPress
Twitter: @SealPress